Welcome to the Peace of Mind Community!

Stay Informed

Stay Informed. Peace of Mind's monthly newsletter includes practices you can use in the classroom and information about events, training and resources. Join the mailing list on our website.

Get Support

If you are new to Peace of Mind, you will find our course "Getting Started with Peace of Mind" very helpful. Visit the Educators page on our website.

Prepare to Teach

You can find links to the materials you need for this curriculum on our website under "Shop."

TeachPeaceofMind.org

Questions? Comments?

We'd love to hear from you!

@PeaceofMindorg   info@TeachPeaceofMind.org

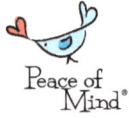

Peace of Mind Core Curriculum for Early Childhood

Peace of Mind Core Curriculum for First and Second Grade

Peace of Mind Core Curriculum for Third Grade

Peace of Mind Curriculum for Fourth and Fifth Grade

Peace of Mind Core Curriculum for Middle School

Henry and Friends Storybook Series

Classroom Tools and Resources

TeachPeaceofMind.org

Peace of Mind Inc, Washington, D.C. 20015
Https://TeachPeaceofMind.org
Copyright 2021 Peace of Mind Inc.

Cover and Interior Design: Schwa Design Group
Illustrations: Gigi Gonyea and Linda Ryden
Photo Credits: Stacy Beck (page 96) and Linda Ryden
Logo: Pittny Creative

ISBN 978-1-7373423-1-1
Library of Congress Control Number: 2021914754
Published 2021

Praise for *Peace of Mind* Curriculum Series

I am astounded by this beautiful curriculum. Linda and her colleagues have created a brilliantly practical guide for teachers, one that understands kids - both how they think, and their imaginative capacities.... This is a model for the classroom of the future.

Jeff Warren, Author and Meditation Teacher

You have done such an outstanding job and this is such a comprehensive curriculum. I am implementing your program...and strongly encouraging my colleagues in our district to do so also.

Cathy Stainbrook, M.A.E, Professional School Counselor

I started using the curriculum and it's wonderful! The lessons are easy to follow and very well thought out. The curriculum fits well with the Mindful Schools training that I did a few years ago. I'm very pleased with my purchase.

Kree Barus, Grade 2 Learning Support Teacher

This is an extraordinary curriculum, at once practical and visionary. The lessons are thoughtfully and meticulously scaffolded as the children are guided step-by-step into an understanding of how their brains work, how to interact with the world with kindness, and how to master themselves. In this age of anxiety, what could be more important or valuable than to teach children at an early age how to interpret and navigate their big emotions, calm themselves, and by extension, each other?

Val Carroll, Early Childhood Arts Integration Educator

We want our children to master their academics but we equally want them to master being good citizens who care about one another and the world at large. The Peace [of Mind] Program does just that. In an age where bullying has become a major problem, the Program is proactive instead of reactive, thereby eliminating some of those problems before they begin.

Jackie Snowden, former Assistant Principal

The importance of teaching kindness, compassion, how to get along, what to do if there is bullying, and how to handle or possibly to avoid conflicts cannot be overstated. The Peace [of Mind] program works. We have been able to see the difference between the students' ability to handle conflicts over the years and we have seen improvement.

Lisa Jensen and Blake Yedwab, Elementary School Teachers

Praise for the *Henry and Friends* Storybook Series

These delightful, captivating books are full of powerful practical methods for kids - and their parents.

Rick Hanson, Ph.D., author of *Resilient, Hardwiring Happiness,* and *Buddha's Brain*

Marleigh is Mindful is a brilliant book of simple and creative mindfulness interventions by an educator who gets children….By framing practice as fundamentally playful, this book brings the benefits of mindfulness and compassion to a new generation. An indispensable toolkit for every classroom and home.

Jeff Warren, Author and Meditation Teacher

In this simple and clear story, Tyaja Uses the Think Test, Linda Ryden offers valuable lessons for our children to bring more clarity, care and thoughtfulness to the power of words.

Oren Jay Sofer, author of *Say What You Mean: A Mindful Approach to Nonviolent Communication*

Linda Ryden's kids' book about Heartfulness practice, Henry is Kind, is bright, fun and engaging, which is wonderful because it means kids will love it. And, the book provides an easy way for teachers and parents to help children understand and enjoy being kind, which means adults will love it too. It is a pleasure to think of the benefits Henry is Kind may bring to children and families.

Sharon Salzberg, author of *Real Happiness and Real Love*

I absolutely adore Sergio Sees the Good. It's a really relatable story for both kids and adults. The science is just right - totally accessible but not "dumbed down." I love the part about the cactus because you show that it's not all bad to focus on the negative stuff and there's a logical reason why evolution didn't do away with it. I think it's also great that you touched on how one can overcome the negativity bias in daily life by noticing and feeling grateful for the "little, good things", even though that feels more effortful.

Dr. Elizabeth Hoffman, Neuroscientist

Contents

Introduction

Supporting students' social and emotional well-being has never been more important. Our kids and educators are coping with anxiety and fear related to the Covid-19 pandemic and facing great uncertainty about returning to school. Before 2020 we knew that we had some students who had experienced some sort of trauma; we know now that all of our students have been through a traumatic experience.

This second edition of the *Peace of Mind Core Curriculum for Grades 1 and 2* includes more trauma-informed practices throughout. We have also included a greater focus on understanding and practicing gratitude which research has shown to be a powerful tool in combating fear and anxiety and building resilience.

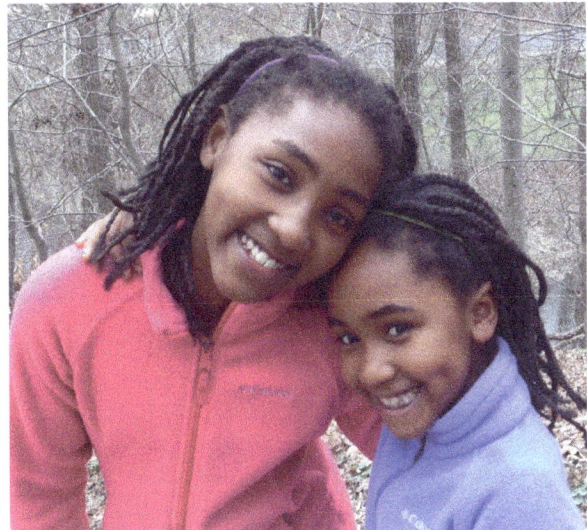

Since we published the first version of this curriculum in 2016, we have continued to learn and develop this program with Linda's students in the dynamic setting of a public school classroom here in Washington D.C.. We have also had the good fortune to hear from many of the educators using the *Peace of Mind Curriculum* at our Annual Conferences and Community of Practice meetings. As a result, you'll find more hands-on activities as well as more movement and pair-sharing incorporated into lessons. We hope you will also enjoy new lessons built around the Peace of Mind story books and several stories to act out written just for the Peace of Mind curriculum.

It has been so exciting to see how educators across the country, and even internationally, have taken up this important work and made this curriculum their own. We hope that you will bring your own experience and skills to bear in adapting the lessons to meet your students' needs in the ways that work best for them and for you.

What *Peace of Mind* offers is more than simply mindfulness practice or social and emotional skills: we offer an integrated, weekly, year-after-year program that teaches skills for life. Combined with your passion and dedication as a teacher, this is a very powerful, transformative combination for our children.

If you find value in teaching *Peace of Mind*, we hope you will share it with your colleagues and friends. Our nonprofit organization, Peace of Mind Inc, exists to be of service to educators who want to bring mindfulness, kindness and conflict resolution to their students. Please help us spread the word!

Thank you for taking up this important work. Your community and your students need what you have to give.

In peace,

Linda and Cheryl July 2021

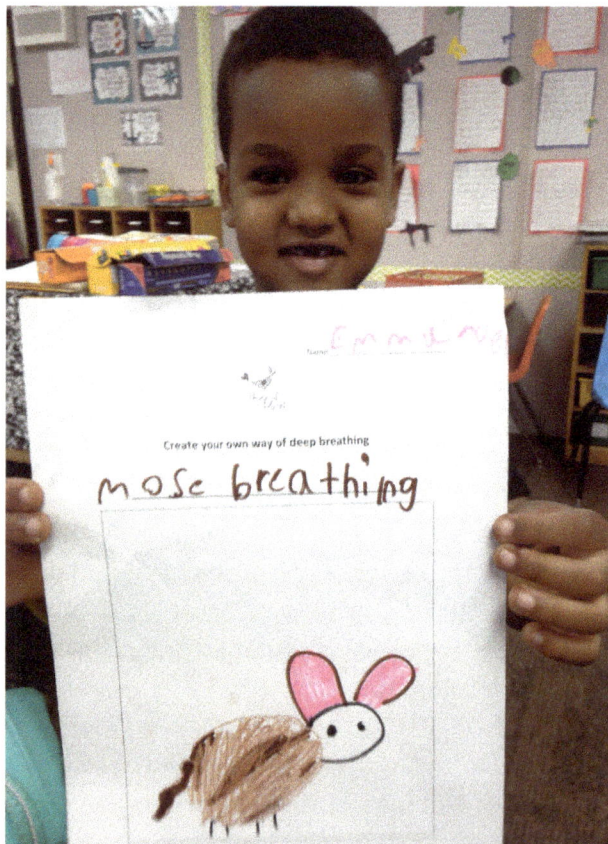

Curriculum Overview

Welcome to the second edition of the *Peace of Mind Core Curriculum for Grades 1 and 2!* All of the Peace of Mind Curricula, including this one, integrate mindfulness practice, brain science, social emotional learning, and conflict resolution for elementary school students.

The Peace of Mind Program helps students develop the skills to notice and manage their emotions, to focus their attention, to practice kindness, empathy and gratitude, to build healthy relationships, and to solve conflicts peacefully - in short, to develop the tools to face life's challenges with compassion and skill.

Teaching the *Peace of Mind Curriculum* weekly over the course of the whole school year, year after year, and integrating elements of *Peace of Mind* into every day, creates positive change in a classroom and, over time, in school climate, moving schools toward kindness and inclusion.

For an overview of the philosophy, history and goals of the Peace of Mind Program, please watch the short video introduction by Peace Teacher and curriculum author Linda Ryden on our website: TeachPeaceofMind.org/videos/.

Curriculum Structure

All *Peace of Mind* curricula include three critical, integrated components:

- Mindfulness
- Brain Science
- Social and Emotional Learning (SEL) with an emphasis on kindness, gratitude and conflict resolution.

Every lesson begins with Mindfulness Practice, and every lesson ends with Kindness Pal practice. Brain science, social emotional learning (SEL) and conflict resolution lessons are particularly effective because they are built upon this foundation.

Mindfulness in this Curriculum is the practice of paying attention to our thoughts, our feelings, and what is happening around us, and putting some space between our reactions and our response. Mindfulness practice might include quietly sitting to focus on breath awareness, practicing mindful listening, noticing how our bodies feel when we have different emotions, engaging in active movement, and more.

Mindfulness practice is becoming more prevalent in schools because research shows that mindfulness training can help to enhance children's attention and focus (Zenner et al., 2014; Zoogman et al. 2015), improve self-control and emotion regulation (Metz et al., 2013), and improve overall social emotional competence including increased empathy, perspective-taking, and emotional control, and less peer-rated aggression (Schonert-Reichl et al., 2014; Schonert-Reichl & Lawlor, 2010).

Brain science is a key ingredient in *Peace of Mind*'s approach. *Peace of Mind* offers students a basic understanding of the roles of the amygdala, the hippocampus and the prefrontal cortex in reacting and responding to stimuli. This knowledge helps students understand how and why we get angry, for example, and how and why practicing mindfulness can help us calm down enough to make a decision that moves us closer to the outcome we'd like to have.

Social and Emotional Learning (SEL) is the process through which we learn to manage emotions; set and achieve positive goals; feel and show empathy for others; establish and manage positive relationships; and make responsible decisions. *(CASEL.org)*

A growing body of research shows that tending to students' social and emotional needs has positive benefits. A meta-analysis of 213 school-based SEL programs with over 270,000 students found that students who received SEL instruction, compared to a control group, showed significantly improved social and emotional skills, attitudes and behavior, and an 11 percent gain in academic achievement. (Durlak et al., 2011).

We are excited about recent research on gratitude which confirms its benefits for social and emotional well-being. According to a white paper produced by the Greater Good Science Center at UC Berkeley for the John Templeton Foundation in 2018, "research suggests that gratitude may be associated with many benefits for individuals, including better physical and psychological health, increased happiness and life satisfaction, decreased materialism, and more."

SEL lessons focus on gratitude and other important topics including kindness, empathy, relationship building, apologizing and using a set of tools to resolve conflicts peacefully.

Ultimately, the goal of *Peace of Mind* is to create a school culture of kindness. Creating a kinder, more positive school climate and dedicating class time for social and emotional learning are two important and evidence-based approaches to bullying prevention (Bradshaw, 2015; O'Brennan & Bradshaw, 2013).

Peace of Mind's goals and lesson structure are aligned with the 5 Core Competencies identified by the Collaborative for Social and Emotional Learning. *(CASEL.org)*

Peace of Mind teaches Mindfulness-based Social and Emotional Learning. We know that mindfulness and SEL both have positive benefits for our students and our schools. But here's what's really exciting: we have learned in over a decade of teaching this work to students that integrating mindfulness with SEL is an even more transformative approach than teaching either mindfulness or SEL on its own.

We can't know what challenges our children will face as they grow, but we have confidence that the combination of these internal and external approaches will give students the ability to meet them with skill and kindness.

Lesson Themes

This curriculum is divided into six sequential units. In these lessons, we are building both self-awareness and regulation and developing our ability to build healthy relationships with others. Lessons help students develop individual awareness of their emotions, develop their own personal mindfulness practices, and practice compassion and kindness toward themselves. Lessons also help students put these lessons to work to practice gratitude for others, to practice kindness toward others, and solve conflicts peacefully. Here's how the units flow:

Unit 1: Mindfulness Foundations (9 lessons)

This unit builds a critical foundation for all the lessons that follow, introducing students to a range of mindfulness practices. Students experience the effects of each practice personally and begin to discern which practices are most helpful to them.

Unit 2: Gratitude (4 lessons)

In this unit, we explore our brain's tendency to focus on the negative and how gratitude practice helps to balance this tendency by focusing on small good things we experience. Through stories, games and activities, students experience this for themselves.

Unit 3: Feelings and Sensations (6 lessons)

In this unit, we explore the embodiment of feelings. When we can notice where feelings begin in our bodies as sensations, it gives us a head start on gaining control over how we respond to them.

Unit 4: Brain Science (5 lessons)

In this unit, we review the functions and interrelatedness of three key parts of our brains: the amygdala, the hippocampus and the prefrontal cortex. Through stories and role plays, students gain powerful insight into themselves and why mindfulness helps us calm down.

Unit 5: Conflict Resolution (5 lessons)

In this unit, we integrate everything we've done until this point. Through stories and role plays, we apply what we've been learning about mindfulness, kindness, empathy, and brain science to the challenge of resolving conflicts peacefully.

Unit 6: Kindness (3 lessons)

We end the curriculum with Kindness. Throughout the year we have been practicing being kind through Kindness Pals and building our classroom community. In this unit, we focus on self-compassion and compassion for others, and end with a Kindness Chain as a final way of connecting with and appreciating each other.

Lesson Sequence

Lessons are designed to be taught in the order in which they are presented. However, we know that in some cases, it may make sense to change the order of lessons to meet your students' needs or to coincide with events in your school community. Please do what you think best meets the needs of your class.

The very first lesson you teach about mindfulness is actually the first step toward peaceful conflict resolution in your classroom. From Week 1, you will be building the foundation that will enable children to solve conflicts with empathy, compassion and skill. Every lesson is a critical piece of the foundation for successful conflict resolution. Without the foundation, the conflict resolution lessons themselves will be less effective.

All of the lessons bear repeating! If you feel your class needs more practice in a certain area, feel free to repeat a lesson, or segment of the lesson, that feels helpful.

Lesson Framework

Each lesson includes the following components:

- **Mindfulness and Mindfulness Helper**

  Mindfulness is the foundation for everything we teach. Reinforcing each child's ability to be a Mindfulness Helper is important. Helping to lead the class in mindfulness practice supports each child in making the practices their own. Leadership of this part of class may be particularly beneficial for children who do not have leadership opportunities in other areas of their lives. You'll find more on the Mindfulness Helper in the next section.

- **Lesson**

  Weekly lessons are designed to be engaging and fun with a balance of listening, discussion and activity. Some lessons focus primarily on introducing a new mindfulness practice; most start with a mindfulness practice as the foundation for topics described above.

- **Storybooks and Skits**

  Many lessons use stories to help engage kids in the ideas and skills being taught. Other lessons engage students in acting out stories to help them practice using the skills and tools they are learning, so that they are available to them when they are really needed.

- **Kindness Pals**

  All lessons close with Kindness Pals. Not only do Kindness Pals give students a way to practice kindness, they are an essential tool for building a positive and inclusive classroom and school community. This practice is described in more detail in the next section.

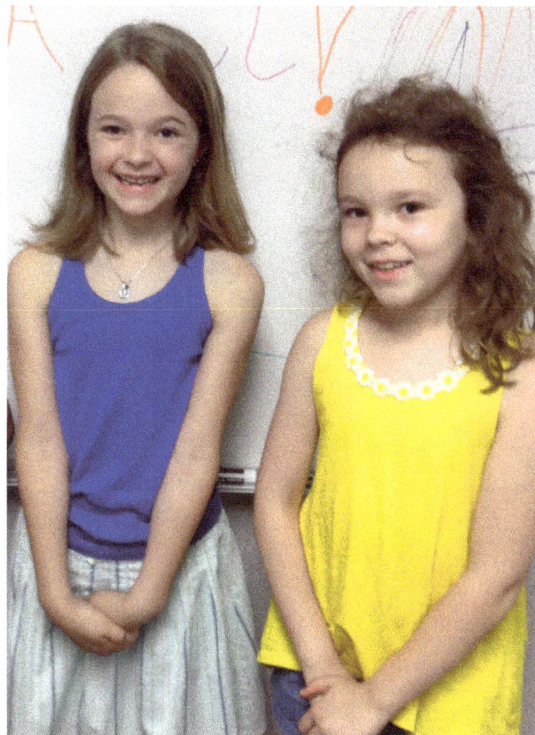

Preparing to Teach

As you begin to review the Curriculum, you will notice that the first paragraph of each lesson offers you an overview of the lesson. All of the lessons offer suggested scripts for you. Please use them as a support, but feel free to teach the lesson in your own words in the way that feels most natural to you.

Once you have read through this guide, it will be helpful to gather materials you will need, spend a little extra time preparing to engage your Mindfulness Helpers and manage Kindness Pals, and take some time for your own mindfulness practice, too. Here's what you will need.

Materials

The list of materials you need to obtain before teaching Peace of Mind is short:

- √ A bell or a chime of some sort that does not have another meaning in your classroom;
- √ Four storybooks. A list follows.

Optional materials include:

- √ A Talking Object, such as a small stuffed animal or bean bag;
- √ A Hoberman Sphere (a breathing ball), available at your local toy store or online;
- √ Brainy the Puppet (available at PeaceofMind.org)

Books and Worksheets

This curriculum includes lessons built around four Peace of Mind storybooks (list below), some original act-out stories contained in the lessons themselves, and some drawing/writing opportunity worksheets. All Worksheet Templates are found in the Resource Section at the end of the Curriculum.

You will need the following storybooks by Linda Ryden. If you do not already have them, you can find them at your favorite online retailer or through TeachPeaceofMind.org/shop/.

Marleigh is Mindful
Rosie's Brain
Sergio Sees the Good
Henry is Kind

Get to Know Two Pillars of Peace of Mind

Before beginning to teach Peace of Mind, please familiarize yourself with the two consistent features of every lesson: the Mindfulness Helper and Kindness Pals.

Mindfulness Helper

An important component of the mindfulness portion of the curriculum is a Mindfulness Helper. The Mindfulness Helper is a student who leads the class in mindful breathing to prepare for the lesson of the day. The Mindfulness Helper concept is introduced after basic ideas of mindful bodies, mindful listening, and mindful breathing have been established.

Where "Mindfulness Helper" is indicated you may follow these steps or create your own ritual. The placement of the steps is indicated in each lesson that includes a Mindfulness Helper (MH).

- The teacher consults their alphabetical roll list and chooses a student to be the Mindfulness Helper for the day.

- The teacher encourages the class to offer sign language applause for the person who is chosen that day.

- The MH comes to the front of the class and sits next to the teacher on a chair or on the floor if you are sitting in a circle.

- With the teacher's help the MH says slowly, "Let's get into our mindful bodies…. Let's close our eyes or look down. … Let's take three deep breaths." Always offer the students a choice about keeping their eyes open or closed.

- At this point the teacher will lead the rest of the mindfulness practice as instructed in the lesson.

- The MH rings the bell when the mindfulness practice is complete.

- The teacher then asks the MH to return to their seat.

You will need to help younger students to remember what to say at the beginning of the year. Repeating the same words each class is important to help students develop a routine to help them begin to practice on their own.

Kindness Pals

Kindness Pals is a very popular activity that achieves several goals:

- To remind the children to make kindness part of their daily lives. Doing kind things for their Kindness Pals spills over into their treatment of others.

- To develop the habit of treating people with kindness through regular practice.

- To give children opportunities to get to know each other and to connect with others whom they might not have gotten along with in the past or whom they think they just don't like.

Here is how it works:

- Each week you assign each student one Kindness Pal. You can pair up the children in advance using the Kindness Pals template (see the Resource Section).

- When children receive the names of their Kindness Pals, emphasize that both pals must say "Okay." This is very important. This lets the teacher know that they have heard their assignment and that they know who their Kindness Pals are. Please practice this with your class.

- Please let the class know that this is not a time for them to let the teacher or the class know how they feel about having that Kindness Pal. This avoids hurt feelings and also offers multiple chances to remind the children that they have the power to be kind and the power to hurt people's feelings. It all depends on their choices. This is a powerful lesson.

- Explain to the students that they will each receive one Kindness Pal each week. It is their job to do nice things for their assigned Kindness Pals for the whole week. Some examples of kind behavior might be to get a Pal's snack, stack their chair, or play together at recess.

- The following week, allow children to talk about what they did for their Pal, allowing about 5 minutes for this sharing.

- Optional: Use some sort of Taking Object (a stuffed animal or squishy ball) for the sharing. Toss the object to the first speaker and remind everyone that the person holding the object gets to talk and the rest of us get to listen.

- Kindness Pals sharing time is a perfect time to practice mindful listening. It's important to demonstrate how we listen mindfully with our whole bodies. Later in the year you might start to let a child lead the sharing and, if you're using one, toss the talking object to the speakers. They love that.

- Then, assign new Kindness Pals for the week ahead.

Especially at the beginning of the year it can help the children remember who their Kindness Pal is if you give them a little chance to chat or greet each other in a friendly way with a high five or friendly words. Any time that you have extra time at the end of a lesson you can give the children an opportunity to chat with their Kindness Pal about some aspect of the lesson or to share their plans for the weekend, for example.

If you are a classroom teacher, you can use Kindness Pals as partners, field trip buddies, and so on. You might allow time for kids to make cards or other things for their Kindness Pal. If you are a counselor or another teacher visiting a classroom, you can talk to the classroom teacher about integrating Kindness Pals into their routine as well as ways to encourage the children to practice kindness.

If you are in a hybrid or virtual setting you might have your students send messages to each other in the chat or make little videos saying hello to each other.

Mindfulness for Yourself

All that's left is to prepare yourself.

It is so important to establish your own mindfulness practice before you attempt to teach it to your students. Just as you would never try to teach Spanish before you learned the language yourself, it is important to begin your own mindfulness practice before bringing these simple but transformative skills to your students. You don't have to be an expert in mindfulness, but it is important to join your students on the journey.

There are so many great resources to help you get started. Ten Percent Happier, Calm and Headspace are secular, simple, step-by-step mindfulness program apps. There are also dozens of books to help you get started. There are more resources listed in the Resources section.

The Peace of Mind online courses are also designed to help you get started in teaching this Curriculum. You can find out more about them at TeachPeaceofMind.org/Educators.

Still have questions?

After reading the introductory material here, you may still find you have questions or feel you need more support.

We have created a two-hour online course just for you called "Getting Started with Peace of Mind." You can find a link to the course in the Educators section of our website: TeachPeaceofMind.org.

Feel free to check in with us directly anytime too. Info@TeachPeaceofMind.org

I think Peace class is very important because it could help bullies calm down and not bully and it will help people calm down in tough situations.

- Peace of Mind Student at Lafayette Elementary School, Washington

Curriculum At-a-Glance

Unit 1 – *Mindfulness Foundations*			
Week	**Mindfulness Skill**	**Lesson Objective(s)**	**Materials for Lessons**
			These materials are needed for every lesson: Kindness Pals list, bell or chime, optional talking object
1. Experiencing Mindfulness	Mindful Listening	Experience mindfulness through our senses. Establish kindness practice.	Kindness Pals Worksheet
2. Animal Breaths	Create Your Own	Introduce the concept of mindfulness and create the foundation for mindfulness practice. Have fun with mindful breathing. Help students experience creating their mindfulness practice. Practice kindness.	Animal Breaths Worksheet
3. Meet Marleigh and Tummy Breaths	Tummy Breaths	Teach basic skills of mindfulness practice. Practice kindness.	*Marleigh is Mindful* Book. A Hoberman Sphere (optional).
4. Take Five Breathing	Take 5 Breathing	Practice using breathing to help calm down. Introduce Mindfulness Helper. Practice kindness.	Copies of the Take 5 Worksheet. *Marleigh is Mindful* Book.
5. Mindful Seeing	Take 5 Review and Mindful Seeing	Practice noticing details. Practice focusing on one thing. Practice kindness.	*Marleigh is Mindful* Book.
6. Mindful Listening Walk	Take 5 Review and Mindful Listening	Use our senses to notice sights and sounds around us. Practice kindness.	
7. Heartfulness	Heartfulness	Using the practice of thinking kind thoughts to increase feelings of compassion and empathy for yourself and others. Practice kindness.	*Marleigh is Mindful* Book. Heartfulness Worksheet.

Week	Mindfulness Skill	Lesson Objective(s)	Materials for Lessons
8. Moving Mindfully	Candle Breaths, Mirror Game, and Freeze Dancing	Learn how Mindful Movements help to connect our bodies and minds and heighten our sense of control of our bodies. Practice Candle Breaths. Practice kindness.	*Marleigh is Mindful* Book. Music for Freeze Dancing.
9. Wave Breathing	Wave Breathing and Student Creations	Experiment with deep breathing. Practice kindness.	*Marleigh is Mindful* Book. "Create Your Own Way of Breathing" Worksheet.
Unit 2 – Gratitude			
10. Feeling Grateful	Gravity Hands and Gratitude Practice	Learn to develop a gratitude practice. Introduce Gravity Hands. Practice kindness.	*Marleigh is Mindful* book. Listen to "Tell Me Something Good" by Chaka Kahn. Copies of the "I am grateful for…" Worksheet.
11. Sergio Sees the Good	Cup of Gratitude	Learn about Negativity Bias and how we can help our brains remember the little good things. Practice kindness.	*Sergio Sees the Good* book.
12. Gratitude Marble Game	Student choice: Take Five, Wave Breathing, or Gravity Hands	Practice training our brain to notice the little good things. Reinforce lessons about Negativity Bias. Practice kindness.	Little cups and marbles or pasta, paperclips, any small things that you have a lot of.
13. Gratefuls Box	Straw Breathing	Practice gratitude by making a Gratefuls Box. Learn about Negativity Bias and how we can help our brains remember the little good things. Practice kindness.	Brown paper bags, clear baggies, empty tissue boxes, whatever you have around. Enough for everyone in your class. Little strips of paper - about 2 inches long. Gratefuls Box Worksheet
Unit 3 – Feelings and Sensations			
14. Mindfulness of Sensations	Noticing Sensations	Practice a new mindfulness exercise. Learn that we can be aware of what is happening in our bodies. Practice kindness.	Kindness Pals Same and Different Worksheet.
15. Mindful Eating	Take 5 Breathing and Mindful Eating	Practice mindful breathing and eating. Apply our mindfulness skills to our everyday lives. Practice kindness.	Enough raisins for all of your class to have one or two. Hand sanitizer.

Week	Mindfulness Skill	Lesson Objective(s)	Materials for Lessons
16. Feelings Game	Flower and Bubble Breaths	Help children name their feelings. Help children to recognize those feelings in others. Practice kindness.	*Marleigh is Mindful* book. Write different emotions on index cards.
17. Finding Your Feelings	Straw Breathing	Help children to locate where they feel emotions in their bodies. Practice kindness.	Copies of the "Finding Your Feelings" Worksheet.
18. Mindful Listening Challenge	Mindful Listening	Practice Mindful Listening. Practice Gratitude. Prace kindness.	Objects that make sounds, such as: scissors, a bell, a jar of marbles, your footsteps. Commonalities Worksheet
19. Visualization	Visualization Practice	Practice mindful breathing. Learn the skill of visualization to calm down and focus. Practice kindness.	*Marleigh is Mindful* book. Copies of the Visualization Worksheet.
Unit 4 – Brain Science			
20. Rosie's Brain	Student choice: Take Five, Wave Breathing, or Gravity Hands	Learn three parts of your brain. Practice kindness.	*Rosie's Brain* book. Brainy the Puppet (optional).
21. Learn About Your Amygdala with Brainy	Take 5 Breathing	Learn about how the Amygdala operates. Practice kindness.	Copies of the Amygdala Worksheet. Review video of Dr. Daniel Siegel's Model of the Brain. Diagram of the brain.
22. Learn About Your PFC with Brainy	Student choice: Take Five, Wave Breathing, or Gravity Hands	Learn about the role of the Prefrontal Cortex. Practice kindness.	Brainy the Puppet (optional).
23. Learn about your Hippocampus with Miss Pickles	Blooming Breaths	Learn about the Hippocampus. Practice gratitude. Practice kindness.	*Marleigh is Mindful* book. Brainy the Puppet (optional).
24. Jonah Flips His Lid	Take 5 Breathing and Wave Breathing	Learn about using Mindful Breathing to help when you flip your lid. Practice kindness.	Brainy the Puppet (optional).

Unit 5 – Conflict Resolution			
Week	**Mindfulness Skill**	**Lesson Objective(s)**	**Materials for Lessons**
25. Learn About Conflict with Daisy and Cactus	Color Breaths	Practice Mindful Breathing and noticing thoughts. Introduce the word "conflict". Practice kindness.	Brainy the Puppet (optional).
26. The Conflict Escalator	Blooming Breaths	Help children understand there is nothing but TROUBLE at the top of the conflict escalator. Practice kindness.	Brainy the Puppet (optional). Review *The Story of Dorothy and Natalie* in the lesson. Copies of the Conflict Escalator Worksheet.
27. The Guinea Pig Conflict	Squeeze and Release	Reinforce the concept of the conflict escalator. Practice kindness.	Brainy the Puppet (optional). Copies of the Conflict Escalator Worksheet. Review *The Guinea Pig Conflict* story in lesson.
28. Working it out with Louise and Jack	Squeeze and Release	Learn one method of conflict resolution. Practice kindness.	Brainy the Puppet (optional). Review *The Story of Louise and Jack* in the lesson. Jack and Louise Worksheet.
29. Working it out with Jahiem and Avi	Gravity Hands	Practice Gravity Hands. Practice working out conflicts peacefully. Practice kindness.	Brainy the Puppet (optional). Review *The Story of Jahiem and Avi* in the lesson. Jahiem and Avi Worksheet.
Unit 6 – Kindness			
30. Henry is Kind	Heartfulness	Help the children get into the habit of doing kind things. Notice the good feelings that come from showing kindness to others. Practice Heartfulness.	*Henry is Kind* Book. Chart paper for making an Anchor Chart. Sticky notes with hearts drawn on them. Kind to Me Worksheet.
31. Gratitude Cards	Heartfulness	Practice mindful gratitude. Encourage the children to appreciate the kindness of the people around them and to practice expressing that gratitude.	Enough paper folded in half like a card for all of the school staff you will thank, crayons or markers. Make sure to include office staff, custodians, school resource officers, and so on.
32. The Kindness Chain	Heartfulness	Practice mindful breathing. Illustrate the power of words to start a chain of kindness. Make a kindness chain. Practice kindness.	

Teaching *Peace of Mind* in First and Second Grade

The following lessons for first and second graders focus on using their senses, moving their bodies, noticing their feelings, understanding how their own minds work, and caring for and working out conflicts with others.

Introducing mindfulness to young children is actually very easy because they seem to instinctively understand the concept. It is not necessary to define "mindfulness" formally for them; this practice names something that they are already doing.

Anger, frustration and other big emotions are part of everyday life for young children and often lead to conflict. Mindfulness practice can help children recognize when they are getting angry or experiencing another big emotion, and to assist them in staying calm. The goal of mindfulness is not to help children bury or deny their emotions. We hope to help kids learn how to manage and deal with their emotions in a way that is helpful to them.

Kindness is a skill that can be practiced and learned. The goal of the Social and Emotional Learning lessons is to help children use kindness, empathy and gratitude to build strong, healthy relationships with friends and family.

> *Even if I come to Peace class sad or not feeling well or just in a bad mood, I always become very calm and happy by the end… everything about Peace class is wonderful. I love it!!*
>
> - Peace of Mind student

Goals and Expectations

Peace of Mind's goals for first and second graders are listed below. You'll notice that each goal starts with "Begin to." *The Peace of Mind* curriculum is planting seeds of mindfulness and compassion. These seeds grow and mature inside a student's mind and heart, positively affecting the way a person sees the world and operates within it. For some students, the outward positive effects are manifested quickly and clearly. For other students, it may take more time, and the outward signs of change may be subtle. All that we expect of students is to try to practice the skills in this curriculum as often as they can. Just to try.

Classroom Management

Some kids have a much easier time sitting quietly than others. Keep your expectations reasonable. Sometimes the kid who is sitting with his eyes wide open, legs jiggling, and fiddling with a pencil—but not talking—during mindfulness practice is doing his very best and is benefiting greatly from the effort. That's okay. The exercises in this curriculum are for the benefit of the children and, as long as they are not preventing other children from practicing, a little wiggling around is okay.

Try to put the guidelines in positive language such as "As long as you follow the directions you can continue to play the game." This can be much more effective than the more traditional way of saying, "If you don't follow the rules you can't play." Many children react defiantly to orders like that but are perfectly happy to follow the rules when they are stated in a more neutral way.

Trauma Sensitive Teaching

One important area of growth in our field is in the area of trauma-sensitive mindfulness teaching. While mindfulness can be tremendously helpful for most people, for some, certain practices may trigger traumatic responses. These responses might range from discomfort and twitchiness to intense memories of a traumatic event. As teachers, our role is to notice our children's responses, to remind them that they always have a choice about whether to do a certain practice or not, to offer an alternative, to be flexible, and to seek help when we feel out of our depth.

Here are a few guidelines that we hope will be helpful to you in your teaching:

- Offering choice is essential.
- Be flexible. Suggest different points of focus, invite open or closed eyes, and allow some flexibility with body position and movement, as long as adaptations for one child do not compromise the ability of other children to practice.
- Reassure children they can stop a practice anytime, or choose another practice as long as it doesn't interfere with anyone else's practice.
- Notice what is happening for your students as they practice. Check in with children who seem uncomfortable, and offer a quiet alternative.
- You know your students best. Read over the skits and stories with your students in mind. Feel free to change any language or scenarios that might not be relevant or appropriate. Feel free to change the language - changing parent to guardian for example - or in any other way that will make the stories more accessible and comfortable for your students.
- Seek additional help if needed.

We encourage you to learn more about this area. Here are two excellent resources: *Trauma-Sensitive Mindfulness: Practices for Safe and Transformative Healing* by David Treleaven and *The Trauma Sensitive Classroom* by Patricia Jennings.

Differentiation

Modeling what you teach

Students will take their cues from you. As we've already said, it is so important to establish your own mindfulness practice before you attempt to teach it to your students, and to continue to be open to learning along with your students. You don't have to be an expert in mindfulness but it is important to join your students on the journey.

You may have already found resources that support you in teaching the *Peace of Mind Curriculum*. If not, there are a few good ones listed in the Resource area of the Appendix. and in the Educator section of the *Peace of Mind website* TeachPeaceofMind.org

Goals for First and Second Grade

- Begin to understand how to listen, speak, act, and move mindfully.
- Begin to understand how some important parts of the brain work.
- Begin to develop the habit of being kind.
- Begin to practice gratitude.
- Begin to acquire a basic understanding of conflict and an awareness of relevant choices.
- Begin to be able to calm oneself and focus one's attention.

I think Peace of Mind is important because it helps people if they are upset; they know how to calm down to talk it out… It also makes school more enjoyable.

- Peace of Mind student

t

Unit 1:
Lessons

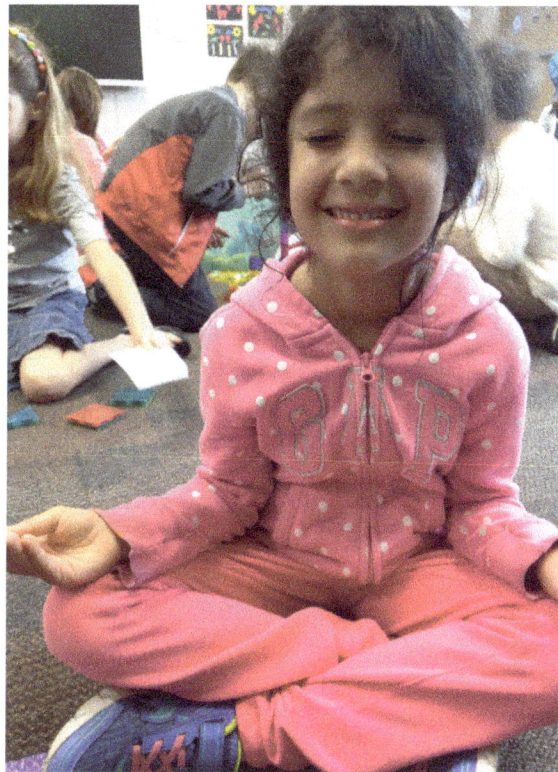

Week 1
Experiencing Mindfulness; Kindness Pals

MINDFULNESS PRACTICE: Mindful Listening

OBJECTIVES: Experience mindfulness through our senses.

                         Establish a kindness practice.

PREPARE: A bell or chime

                         My Kindness Pal Worksheet

                         Your Kindness Pals list (see Resource Section)

Welcome to Peace of Mind! The Mindfulness Practices that make up the first unit of this curriculum are the critical foundation for the SEL, Brain Science and Conflict Resolution lessons that follow. In our first lesson today, we will introduce the practice of Mindful Listening, the first of many practices we will explore. This practice helps to calm the nervous system and to direct our attention to where we want to focus. We will also introduce an important pillar of the Peace of Mind Curriculum: Kindness Pals. Let's dive in!

Mindfulness Practice

1. Introduce the lesson

Say: *Today we are going to start learning about something new together. It's called mindfulness.*

Mindfulness is fun because anyone can do it, you can do it anywhere, and you have everything you need to do it right in your own body. You have probably tried it already and didn't even know it.

Mindfulness is about noticing things. Sometimes we'll notice things by listening or seeing or even by sitting quietly with our eyes closed. Sometimes we'll be moving, and sometimes we'll be eating!

Are you ready to start?

The first thing we are going to do is listen.

I'd like you to close or cover your eyes and I'm going to set a timer for thirty seconds. During that time I want you to count inside your mind, not out loud, how many different sounds you hear.

Try not to make any sounds yourself. Just sit really still and count the sounds you hear. You might have to listen really hard to hear things. Ready? Close or cover your eyes. Okay, let's start listening now…

Wait about thirty seconds or longer if they seem to have an easy time staying still. You might subtly add some sounds (chair squeaking, foot-steps, keys softly jingling, etc.) if the room is really quiet.

Say: *Now let's open our eyes.*

2. Discuss.

Leave plenty of time for sharing. You might use these kinds of questions to frame a discussion:

- Who would like to tell us about a sound that you heard?
- How did you know it was a door squeaking if you couldn't see the door?

Try to hear from everyone, even if they are sharing about a sound that had already been mentioned.

If you are short on time, have them share with an elbow partner instead.

3. Make connections.

Conclude this portion of the lesson by encouraging students to use mindful listening at home.

Say:

Isn't it interesting how many different sounds we could hear?

All of these sounds were all around us and yet we weren't paying attention to them.

This is something you can try anytime—when you are at home, or in the car, or outside on the playground. Just stop and take a moment to do some mindful listening.

Kindness Pals

Introduce Kindness Pals by saying:

Now we are going to start something called Kindness Pals. Every time we meet I am going to give you a Kindness Pal. It will be a different person in your class each time.

I'm going to ask you to do something kind for this person between now and the next time we meet. It can be something small like stacking her chair or something bigger like drawing him a picture or making her a card or playing with your Pal at recess. You can even do more than one thing.

Can you think of other kind things you could do for your Kindness Pal?

Give students time to share.

Say:

I have one very important rule about Kindness Pals. Since the whole point of Kindness Pals is to help us practice being kind, I want to make sure that we start out with kindness. So, when I tell you who your Kindness Pal is going to be, I want you to say "okay" in a friendly way. Let's try that all together: "Okay!"

When I tell you who your Kindness Pal is, you might feel really happy and excited. Maybe your Kindness Pal is already your really good friend and it will be really easy to be kind to them.

But sometimes when I tell you who your Kindness Pal is, you might feel differently. You might feel a little nervous or shy. And that's fine. Any way that you feel is fine. But in that moment I want you to try really hard to be kind to your Pal and say a friendly "Okay!" That way your Pal will know that you are ready to show them some kindness.

You don't have to become friends with your Pal (although you might) and you don't even have to like your Pal. All I'm asking you to do is to find some way to be kind to them this week.

When we meet next time I'm going to ask you to try to remember something that you did for your Kindness Pal and share it with the class. Are you ready to find out who your Kindness Pal is?

Read through the list, saying, for example: "Rosie and Henry are Kindness Pals."

Wait for the "Okay" before moving on.

Say: *Now that you know who your Kindness Pal is, we're going to find out a little more about them. Who can think of a question that we could ask our Kindness Pal?*

Listen to students' suggestions. They might suggest asking about their favorite color or favorite food or sport.

Choose three questions.

Ask the students to sit with their Kindness Pals and have a little chat.

Share. If you have time, you can come back together as a group and ask them to share something that they learned about their Kindness Pals. This exercise is a great way to practice Mindful Listening and help them to develop an interest in others.

Say: *Okay, so now we've gotten to know our Kindness Pal a little better.*

Activity: *Now we're going to do a little drawing. On the My Kindness Pal Worksheet you can draw a picture of your Kindness Pal and then choose a few things that you could do for them this week.*

> *NOTE: This is a worksheet that you can use every week if you'd like.*

I can't wait until next time when we get to hear about the kind things you did for your Pal. Have fun!

Closing Words: *Let's have a nice quiet moment with the bell. You can close your eyes or leave them open, but let's sit quietly and listen to the bell. If you want to, you can think about your new Kindness Pal and imagine yourself doing something kind for them.*

Ring the bell or chime. *Thanks for a great class, everyone.*

Week 2
Animal Breaths

MINDFULNESS PRACTICE: Animal Breaths, Mindful Bodies

OBJECTIVES:
Introduce the concept of mindfulness and create the foundation for mindfulness practice.

Have fun with mindful breathing.

Students create their own mindfulness practices.

Practice kindness.

PREPARE:
A bell or chime

Animal Breaths Worksheet

Your Kindness Pals list

Optional: Something to use as a Talking Object—this could be a stuffed animal or something else soft that you can easily pass around the room

Today we introduce the concept of Animal Breaths and invite students to create their own mindful breathing practices. Our goal is to help students experience mindfulness as their own practice from the very beginning. You might notice that we aren't offering the students definitions of mindfulness. Instead, we are inviting them to experience it and to feel the benefits for themselves. We will introduce several more practices in this unit, not with the goal of mastering them all, but of allowing students to have enough to choose from that they will find one that works best for them.

Mindfulness Practice

1. **Introduce the lesson.**

   You might say: *Last time we had fun practicing paying attention to sounds. Today we're going to have some fun making up ways to take deep breaths. Taking deep breaths is a big part of mindfulness. Deep breaths can help us to calm down when we get mad or upset and it feels good. First let's get into our Mindful Bodies!*

2. Introduce the concept of Mindful Bodies.

Say: *Another thing that we pay attention to when we do mindfulness is our bodies. Today we are going to try something called Mindful Bodies. This is the way we are going to sit when we practice being mindful. Sitting up a little bit straighter and keeping our bodies a little bit still can help us to pay attention to things like sounds or our breath.*

One fun way to get into your Mindful Body is to pretend that you have a zipper that goes from your belly button to your chin. You can pretend to zip up your zipper and straighten your back as you go up. When you get to the top you can unzip a little bit until you find a nice, comfortable position that makes you feel a little more awake and ready.

Offer Choice about what to do with your eyes. *Another part of being in your Mindful Body is deciding what to do with your eyes. Closing your eyes can help you to focus on things like sounds or your breath. If you don't feel comfortable closing your eyes, you could just decide to look down into your lap. It's up to you!*

Practice getting into mindful bodies in this way a few times.

Prompt the students to feel the difference between the way we normally sit and the way we sit when we are ready to be mindful.

NOTE FROM LINDA: *Don't stress about having all kids get into picture perfect mindful bodies! Very few kids will actually stay in their mindful bodies for long if at all. Inviting them to get into their Mindful Bodies is a helpful way to make a transition into what you are doing and to help them practice for the future. If a child is sitting with their eyes wide open, that's fine. I usually ask the kids not to look at each other to give everyone a little privacy. For some kids closing their eyes can be triggering so it's very important to give kids plenty of options and leeway.*

3. Practice mindful listening.

Say: *Now let's practice some mindful listening like we did yesterday.*

Say: *I'm going to ring this bell (or chime or whatever you have). I'll ring it one time while you are looking at it and then we'll try to listen to it with our eyes closed or looking down.*

Ring the bell for the class.

Say: *Okay now let's get into our Mindful Bodies. Zip up and find your comfy, sort of straight position. Close your eyes or look down. This time when I ring the bell try to listen to the whole sound and then raise your hand when you can't hear it anymore.*

Ring the bell again.

Wait for the last student to raise their hand.

Say: *Okay now open your eyes or look up.*

Ask:

- What did you notice about the sound?
- Were you able to keep your mind focused on the sound? Or did your mind wander to think about something else?
- Did being in your Mindful Body help you to pay attention to the sound?

Conclude by saying: *If your mind wandered away instead of listening to the bell don't worry! That is perfectly normal. That's what minds do sometimes. The more we practice, the easier it will be to stay focused on the sound.*

Lesson: Fun with Mindful Breathing

1. Make up your own Animal Breath

The purpose of this lesson is to get kids used to taking these deep breaths, bring movement into the class, and to have fun. This will lay the foundation for other kinds of mindfulness practices and will give the kids a sense of ownership over their own mindfulness practice in the future.

You might say: *Like I said earlier, one of the best ways to help us to calm down when we get mad or frustrated is to take some deep breaths. There are lots of ways to do this. Let's see what we can make up right now!*

Let's start by thinking about animals. Let's make up some Animal Breaths. We could do Butterfly Breaths by pretending that we are slowly flapping our wings up and down.

Demonstrate by slowly moving your arms up and down like butterfly wings.

Say*: When we breathe in we can flap our arms up and when we breathe out we can flap our arms down. Let's try that a few times. Let's pretend we are a butterfly moving in slow motion and do it really slowly and gently.*

Ask*:* Can you think of another Animal Breath?

Invite the kids to create their own Animal Breaths and ask a few to share. Encourage everybody to try each idea.

2.   Draw a picture of your Animal Breathing Idea

Hand out copies of the Animal Breaths Worksheet.

Invite the students to draw a picture of their own Animal Breath.

Sending these worksheets home provides a valuable family connection to what children are learning in class.

Kindness Pals

Following is a suggested structure and script for Kindness Pals that you can use each week if you like.

The talking object is optional. For some classes this can be a helpful way of keeping the other kids focused on the speaker. If it's a distraction or not necessary for your group, feel free not to use it.

Don't worry if the kids don't remember to do anything for their Kindness Pal. This might take practice and some gentle reminders.

You might begin by saying: *Last time we met I gave you a Kindness Pal and asked you to do something kind for them. Did anybody remember to do something for their Pal?*

Who would like to share what you did?

I'm going to [pass the talking object to/ call on] someone who is ready to share.

If using the talking object, say: *When you are holding the talking object, it is your turn to share. If you are not holding the talking object, it is your turn to listen.*

If you are not using the talking object, be sure to remind your students to really listen to each other. This is such an important life skill and there are so many opportunities to practice it in these lessons.

Pass the object to someone or call on someone to speak, and then pass the turn to their Kindness Pal who can either share what they did, or they can say "thank you" to their Pal. This little practice helps the children to develop a sense of gratitude for little kindnesses.

Assign new Kindness Pals after they are finished sharing. See the instructions in the "How To Use This Curriculum" section above.

Assign new Kindness Pals after they are finished sharing. See the instructions in the "How To Use This Curriculum" section above.

If you have time, you can give them time for a Kindness Pal chat like they had in Lesson 1.

Closing Words: *Our time is up for today. Let's have a nice quiet moment with the bell. You can close your eyes or leave them open, but let's sit quietly and listen to the bell. If you want to, you can think about your new Kindness Pal and imagine yourself doing something kind for them.*

Ring the bell or chime. *Thanks for a great class, everyone.*

If you are a classroom teacher, you might consider making Kindness Pals time a regular part of the weekly schedule by setting aside a little time each week for kids to make their Pal a card or drawing or to spend a little time together. You can assign kids to work with Kindness Pals or read together or sit together on field trips.

Week 3
Meet Marleigh and Tummy Breaths

MINDFULNESS PRACTICE: Tummy Breaths

OBJECTIVES: Teach the basic skills of mindful breathing practice.

Practice kindness.

PREPARE: A bell or chime

Your Kindness Pals list

Marleigh is Mindful by Linda Ryden

Optional: Talking Object

Optional: A Hoberman Sphere

Marleigh is Mindful is a book that I wrote that teaches children how to use mindfulness practices to help them deal with big emotions. The book is an excellent companion to this curriculum and offers a way to extend, integrate and reinforce lessons in the curriculum. We have included practices from the book in this lesson and several others. We encourage you to have it on your bookshelf for your students to look through on their own.

Mindfulness Practice

1. **Explain more about mindful breathing.**

    You might say:

    Today we are going to talk some more about breathing. Breathing is something you do all day and night, every day, but you hardly ever think about it. When are some times that you might be more aware or mindful of your breath?

    Allow children to answer. Their responses will likely be along the lines of: when you are "out of breath" after a big run, when you are angry and breathing hard, and so on.

    Choose a couple of students (or ask all of them) to run quickly in place for 30 seconds. Ask them to notice how they are breathing when they are finished.

Ask students to demonstrate:

- How do you breathe when you are angry?
- What happens to your breath when you are surprised? (gasp!)

2. Lead the class in a mindful breathing exercise.

You might say:

Today we are going to be mindful of our breathing. First let's get into our mindful bodies. Let's keep our eyes open for now.

Put one hand on your belly and see what you notice. Does your belly go in and out when you breathe? Stay there and notice what that feels like for a few breaths.

Now move your hand to your chest. What do you notice here?

Now make your hand like a little cup under your nose. Can you feel the breath going in and out? Do you notice that the breath feels a little bit cooler going in and a little bit warmer going out?

Now I'd like you to choose one of those three places where we could feel our breath. Choose the place where you could feel your breath the most.

Now Let's close our eyes or look down. We are going to try to focus our minds on our breath for a few seconds. See if you notice if all of your breaths feel the same or if some are different.

When time is up, you might say:

Now let's open our eyes and share what we felt.

Leave plenty of time for the children to share what they felt.

3. IntroduceTummy Breaths

Say: *Now we are going to try doing something called Tummy Breaths.*

Tummy breaths are a great way to help you calm down, if you are really mad, angry, sad or nervous. Raise your hand if you have ever been really mad or angry. What does that feel like?

Take a few answers.

What does your breath feel like when you are angry?

Take a few answers.

Say: *We have all felt angry before. Taking a few deep tummy breaths can really help you feel like yourself again. And it's pretty easy once you get the hang of it! First watch me.*

Place your hands on your belly and take a deep breath in through your nose and expand your belly as you breathe in. Make it a little exaggerated so that they can see it. Exhale through your mouth and let it go back toward your spine. Do this a few times.

Say: *What did you notice about the way I was breathing? Did you see how my tummy went out when I breathed in and went back in when I breathed out?*

It's like I have a little balloon in my belly. When I breathe in I am filling the balloon full of air. When I breathe out I am emptying the balloon.

Let's get into our mindful bodies and try it together. Put your hands on your belly and take a deep breath in through your nose and try to imagine that you are filling the little balloon inside your belly with air.

Now breathe out slowly and gently through your mouth and imagine that you are emptying the balloon. Try that several times slowly and gently

4. **Optional: Introduce the Breathing Ball.**

    If you have the Hoberman Sphere and want to give the kids a chance to try it it can be helpful. If not you can skip to the next section.

    Use the Hoberman Sphere to demonstrate the motion of breathing.

    You might say: *Let's think about this in a different way. Imagine that this breathing ball is inside of you. When you breathe in, the ball grows.*

Expand the ball.

When you breathe out, the ball shrinks.

Shrink the ball.

Now let's all try it. If we are all very quiet, we can make sure that everyone has a nice quiet moment to practice their breathing.

Pass the ball around so all can try it.

Activity: Tummy Breaths

Say: *Now we're all going to try it. We're going to lie down on the floor and I'm going to give you a little object to put on your belly. Once everybody is ready we are going to place the object on our bellies and then practice slowly moving our bellies up and down when we breathe in and out. It might feel like we are rocking our little object to sleep. We'll try to feel what it's like to take a deep breath into our bellies and then slowly letting the air out and having our bellies go down.*

Encourage the children to practice Tummy Breaths when they go to bed at night with one of their own stuffed animals.

Read and Discuss

Introduce Marleigh is Mindful

Say: *Today I'd like to introduce a new book that we'll be checking in with throughout the year. It's called Marleigh is Mindful. This book includes lots of the mindfulness practices that we'll be learning in this class.*

In the book, a girl named Maura and her sisters use Tummy Breaths. Let's read about why and how they do it.

Read the two pages on Maura and Tummy Breathing.

Ask:

- What problem did Tummy Breathing help Maura with?
- How could Tummy Breathing help you?

Kindness Pals

Say: *Last time we met I gave you a Kindness Pal and asked you to do something kind for them. Did anybody remember to do something for their Pal?*

Who would like to share what you did?

I'm going to [pass the talking object to/call on] someone who is ready to share.

If using the talking object, say: *When you are holding the talking object, it is your turn to share. If you are not holding the talking object, it is your turn to listen.*

If you are not using the talking object, be sure to remind your students to really listen to each other. This is such an important life skill and there are so many opportunities to practice it in these lessons.

Pass the object to someone or call on someone to speak, and then pass the turn to their Kindness Pal who can either share what they did, or they can say "thank you" to their Pal. This little practice helps the children to develop a sense of gratitude for little kindnesses.

Assign new Kindness Pals after they are finished sharing. See the instructions in the "How To Use This Curriculum" section above.

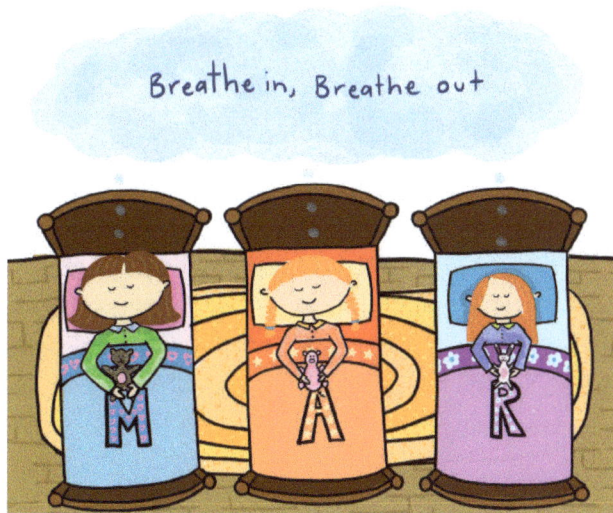

Breathe in, Breathe out

If you have time, you can give them time for a Kindness Pal chat like they had in Lesson 1.

Closing Words: *Let's have a nice quiet moment with the bell. You can close your eyes or leave them open, but let's sit quietly and listen to the bell. If you want to, you can think about your new Kindness Pal and imagine yourself doing something kind for them.*

Ring the bell or chime. *Thanks for a great class, everyone.*

Week 4
Take Five Breathing

MINDFULNESS PRACTICE: Take Five Breathing

OBJECTIVES: Practice using breathing to help calm down.

Introduce the Mindfulness Helper.

Practice kindness.

PREPARE: A bell or chime

Copies of the Take Five worksheet (See Resource section)

Marleigh is Mindful by Linda Ryden

Your Kindness Pals list

Optional: Talking Object

Today we introduce the practice of Take Five Breathing, one of the most beloved practices among Peace of Mind students. Take Five helps students focus on taking five deep breaths while tracing the fingers of one hand. This practice helps children to reconnect with their bodies and to calm the nervous system. It is one of many practices that allow children to take a pause, allowing them to decide how they want to respond in a situation that causes big emotions. We hope you and your students find this practice helpful all year long.

Mindfulness Practice

1. Introduce Take Five breathing

Take Five is a nice way to help children calm themselves down when they are upset or need a break. Here's a sample script to use to introduce the concept.

You might say:

Today we're going to learn another way of using our mindful breathing. Has anyone ever heard someone say "Take Five?"

Take Five means to take a break—usually they mean a five-minute break. We are going to use Take Five in a different way. Hold up your hand like you are going to give someone a high five with your palm facing out and your fingers spread wide.

Now take the index finger of your other hand and trace the outline of your hand. What does it feel like when your finger runs between your fingers? Maybe it's a little tickly?

We're going to do this again, but this time we are going to breathe in when we are tracing up and breathe out when we are tracing down. Starting with your index finger down by your wrist, on the outside of your thumb, trace up your thumb slowly. As you trace up, breathe in, and as you trace down the inside of your thumb, slowly breathe out.

Repeat this motion with all of your fingers until you are back down at your wrist on the outside of your pinky finger. At this point you will have taken five deep breaths.

Take Five is a great way to help you calm down, any time you need a break. See if you can try it a few times this week.

2. **Introduce mindfulness helper.**

> NOTE FROM LINDA: *The Mindfulness Helper becomes quite a coveted position in each class and sometimes the younger children especially are disappointed when it is not their turn. I like to encourage the children to be happy for each other, so I ask them to do sign language applause (wave both hands by the side of your head) when the Mindfulness Helper is chosen and also when the Mindfulness Helper chooses someone to turn on and off the lights.*
>
> *I use this as a teachable moment to help the kids learn that you can choose how you respond to your situation. I remind them that you can choose to be upset every time someone else is chosen, but that means that you will be upset almost every time. Or you can choose to be happy for everyone who is chosen, and then you will be happy every time. Every time I choose the MH I say, "Let's be happy for _____" and for the most part they all join in and feel good. It makes the MH feel good, and that good feeling seems to spread. I also use this method when I choose children to act out the stories*

in the curriculum. This is a good time to remind your students that we often have more than one emotion at the same time and it can be helpful to notice that. We can be happy for someone else and disappointed for ourselves in the same moment.

Say: *Today I am going to ask someone to be my Mindfulness Helper. This person will help to set us up and lead us as we practice our Mindfulness. I am going to go through our class list alphabetically* (or however you choose to do it). *Everyone will have a turn.*

Consult your alphabetical roll list, and choose the first student to be the Mindfulness Helper for the day.

Invite today's Mindfulness Helper (MH) to come to the front of the class to sit next to you on a chair (or next to you on the floor).

Say: *Let's all be happy for* _____. (sign language applause)

Prompt the MH to say: "Let's get into our mindful bodies."

Review what mindful bodies look like.

Prompt the MH to say: "Let's close our eyes or look down."

Say: If you don't feel comfortable closing your eyes you can look straight down into your lap.

> **NOTE:** *Don't worry if some of the children don't close their eyes.*

Prompt the MH to say: "Let's do our Take Five breathing."

Say: *Let's take some nice gentle deep breaths while we trace our hands. When you trace up your finger, breathe in slowly through your nose. When you trace down, breathe slowly out through your mouth. Try to make your breathing so quiet that only you can hear it.*

Now put your hand on your belly and try to make the rest of your body so still and quiet that the only thing that you feel moving is your breath. Notice what you feel there.

Now, let's all listen with our eyes closed or looking down into your lap as the Mindfulness Helper rings the bell. Try to listen to the whole sound of the bell. Open your eyes or look up when you can't hear it anymore.

Ask the MH to ring the bell and return to their seat.

Ask: *How did it feel to do your Take Five breathing?*

> NOTE: *Repeating the same or similar words each class will help to establish a routine that will help the children to practice on their own. With younger students, it will take some time to establish the practice. Be patient with it, and it will become a nice structure for starting the class.*

Read and Discuss

Marleigh is Mindful

Say: *Today let's see who uses Take Five Breathing in Marleigh is Mindful. It's Mason! Let's hear about his experience.*

Read the two pages on Mason and Take Five Breathing.

Ask:

- What problem did Take Five Breathing help Mason with?
- How could Take Five Breathing help you?

Activity: Trace hands on the Take Five worksheet.

Say: *Take Five is a great way to help us to calm down, but we have to remember to use it. Today we're going to make a little poster that you can put up in your room or somewhere at home to help you remember to Take Five.*

Pass out one worksheet to each student.

Have the students trace around one of their hands on the Take Five worksheet. They can decorate their hand in a way that will make them feel happy and peaceful.

Kindness Pals

Do the Kindness Pals activity as before.

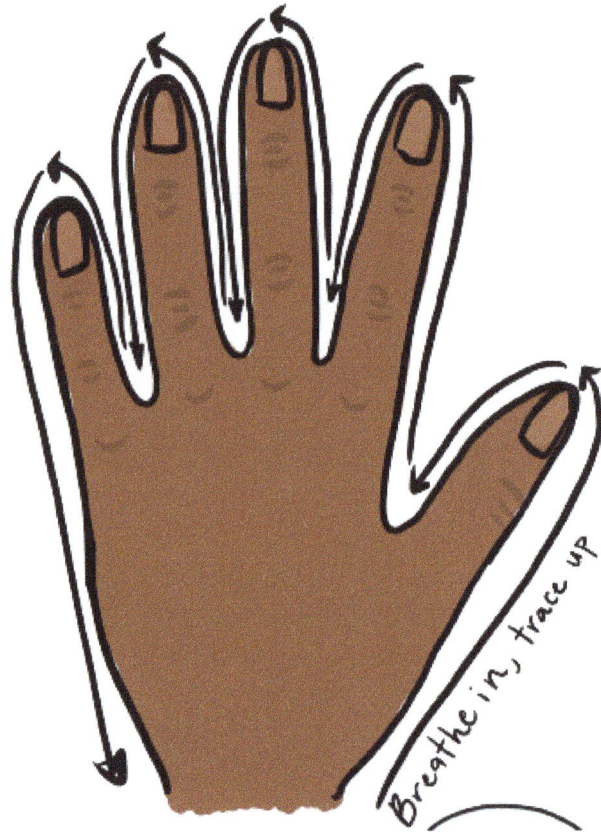

Breathe in, trace up

Closing Words: *Let's have a nice quiet moment with the bell. You can close your eyes or leave them open, but let's sit quietly and listen to the bell. If you want to, you can think about your new Kindness Pal and imagine yourself doing something kind for them.*

Ring the bell or chime. *Thanks for a great class, everyone.*

Week 5
Mindful Seeing

MINDFULNESS PRACTICE: Mindful Seeing and Take Five

OBJECTIVES: Practice noticing details.

Practice focusing on one thing.

Practice kindness.

PREPARE: A bell or chime

Marleigh is Mindful by Linda Ryden

Kindness Pals list

Optional: Talking Object

Today we introduce another type of Mindfulness Practice: Mindful Seeing. This practice helps students focus their attention on what is in their immediate surroundings, including colors, numbers, letters and shapes. Mindful Seeing also offers another way to calm the nervous system when children may be feeling worry or anxiety by helping students turn their attention to what is happening in the moment instead of on what has happened or what might happen. We will begin with a review of Take Five Breathing from last week and play a mindful seeing game called Find the Rainbow.

Mindfulness Practice

1. Remind the class about Take Five breathing

Say: *Just like last time, I am going to ask someone to be my Mindfulness Helper. This person will help to set us up and lead us as we practice our mindfulness. I am going to go through our class list alphabetically (or however you choose to do it). Everyone who wants to will have a turn.*

Invite today's Mindfulness Helper (MH) to come to the front of the class to sit next to you on a chair (or next to you on the floor).

Say: *Let's all be happy for* _____. *(sign language applause)*

Prompt the MH to say: "Let's get into our mindful bodies."

Review what mindful bodies look like.

> **Prompt the MH to say:** "Let's close our eyes or look down."

> **Say:** If you don't feel comfortable closing your eyes you can look straight down into your lap…

> **Prompt the MH to say:** "Let's do our Take Five breathing." Take five deep breaths while tracing your hand.

> *Now, let's all listen as the Mindfulness Helper rings the bell. Try to listen to the whole sound of the bell. Raise your hand and look up or open your eyes when you cannot hear it anymore.*

> **Ask** the MH to ring the bell.

> **Ask** the MH to return to their seat.

> **Ask:** *How did it feel to do your Take Five breathing?*

2. **Practice Mindful Seeing.**

> **Say:** *Today we are going to see what we can notice with our eyes if we are really being mindful, if we are really paying attention. I want you each to choose a color. Raise your hand when you have chosen your color.*

> **Let** some children share their color choice.

> **Say**: *When I say "Go," I'm going to ask you to turn off your voice and walk around the room and count in your head how many times you see your color.*

> *When I ring the bell, it will be time to come back to our seats.*

> **Give them a couple of minutes** to do this activity depending on how long they are able to hold their concentration.

> **Ring** the bell.

> **Share**: You can give them a chance to share with the class how many times they saw their color, or they can share with an elbow partner, or with their Kindness Pal.

> **Say:** Was anybody surprised by how many times you saw your color? Isn't it amazing how many different colors are in this room?

Do you think you could try Mindfully Seeing anywhere else? At home? On your way to school?

> NOTE: *You can try this exercise in a variety of ways. You can have them look for letters, numbers, shapes, etc. It can be a great way to reinforce concepts you are working on in other subjects.*

Read and Discuss

Marleigh is Mindful

Say: *Today let's see who uses Rainbow Breathing in Marleigh is Mindful. It's Charlie and friends! Let's hear about their experience.*

Read the two pages on Charlie and Rainbow Breathing.

Ask*:*

What problem did Rainbow Breathing help Charlie with?

How could Rainbow Breathing help you?

Activity: Find the Rainbow

Say: *Today we're going to learn how to play another mindful seeing game called Find the Rainbow. Find the Rainbow can be a helpful thing to do if you are feeling mad or sad or nervous or frustrated. It can help you to refocus your mind on something other than what is upsetting you.*

Say: *Who can tell us what colors are in the rainbow?*

> NOTE: *You can draw a rainbow or show a picture of a rainbow to illustrate. When you were growing up, you might have learned that the colors of the rainbow were Red, Orange, Yellow, Green, Blue, Indigo and Violet. Some people now say that the colors of the rainbow are Red, Orange, Yellow, Green, Blue and Purple. You can talk about it either way. The accompanying worksheet uses purple instead of indigo and violet.*

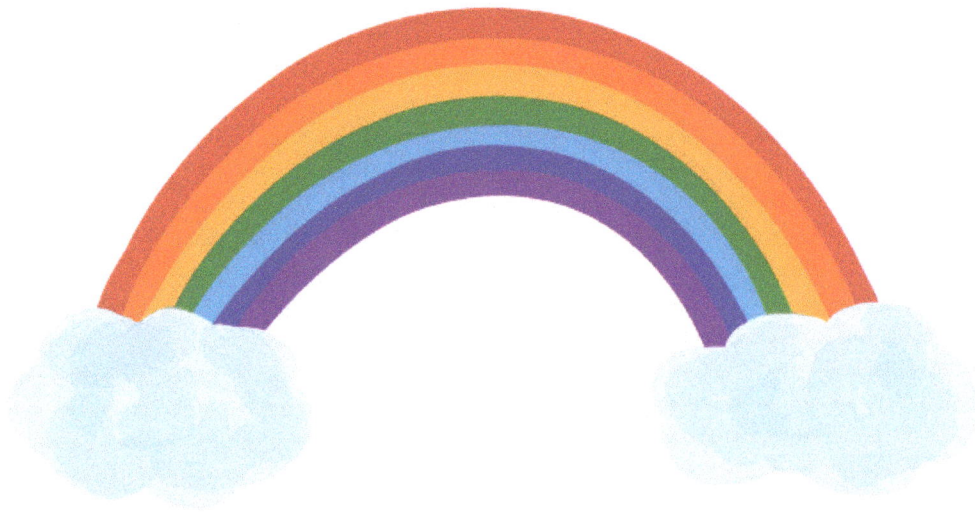

Say: *To play Find the Rainbow you try to find something in the room that matches each color of the rainbow. So you might find a red crayon, an orange backpack, a yellow t-shirt, etc. I'm going to hand out a Find the Rainbow worksheet and you can draw or write about what you found.*

Pass out the Find the Rainbow worksheet . When students are finished, let them share what they found.

Kindness Pals

Do the Kindness Pals activity as before.

Closing Words: *Let's have a nice quiet moment with the bell. You can close your eyes or leave them open, but let's sit quietly and listen to the bell. If you want to, you can think about your new Kindness Pal and imagine yourself doing something kind for him or her.*

Ring the bell or chime. *Thanks for a great class, everyone.*

Week 6
Mindful Listening Walk

MINDFULNESS PRACTICE: Take Five, Mindful Listening Walk

OBJECTIVES: Use our senses to notice sights and sounds around us.

Practice kindness.

PREPARE: A bell or chime

Your Kindness Pals list and Optional Talking Object

Mindfulness Practice

1. Practice Take Five Breathing.

Invite today's Mindfulness Helper (MH) to come to the front of the class to sit next to you on a chair (or next to you on the floor).

Say: *Let's all be happy for _____.* *(sign language applause)*

Say: *Today we are going to practice our Take 5 breathing with our eyes closed.*

Prompt the MH to say: "Let's get into our mindful bodies. Let's close our eyes or look down. Let's take five deep breaths."

Say: *Now with your eyes closed, slowly and gently trace your hand, breathing in as you trace up your finger and breathing out as you trace down. When you are finished you can put your hands in your lap and just breathe.*

Say: *In a moment you will hear the sound of the bell (or chime or whatever you are using). Now, let's all listen with our eyes closed as the Mindfulness Helper rings the bell. Try to listen to the whole sound of the bell. Open your eyes when you cannot hear it anymore.*

Ask the MH to ring the bell when the mindful breathing is complete.

Ask the MH to return to their seat.

2. **Introduce the concept of a Mindful Listening walk.**

   You might say:

   Today we are going to take a mindful walk.

   While we are walking we are going to be very quiet and try to count all of the sounds that we hear.

   When we come back from our walk, we will share all of the different sounds that we hear.

   Ask the children to make a check-list of the sounds they think they might hear. (cars, voices, birds and so on)

3. **Take the class for a walk.**

   It can be a walk outside or a walk through the halls.

   Stop several times during the walk and have the children close their eyes or look down and listen. Let them check their lists at intervals throughout the walk. They can check off the things that they hear as they go along.

4. **Share.**

   When you get back, invite students to share the sounds that they noticed on their walk.

   There are many variations of this walk. You can ask the children to each choose a color and then silently count how many times they see that color on their walk. You can have them work in pairs or teams. You could also have them sit outside or in the classroom and try to draw some of the sounds they hear.

Kindness Pals

   Do the Kindness Pals activity as before.

Closing Words: *Let's have a nice quiet moment with the bell. You can close your eyes or leave them open, but let's sit quietly and listen to the bell. If you want to, you can think about your new Kindness Pal and imagine yourself doing something kind for him or her.*

Ring the bell or chime. *Thanks for a great class, everyone.*

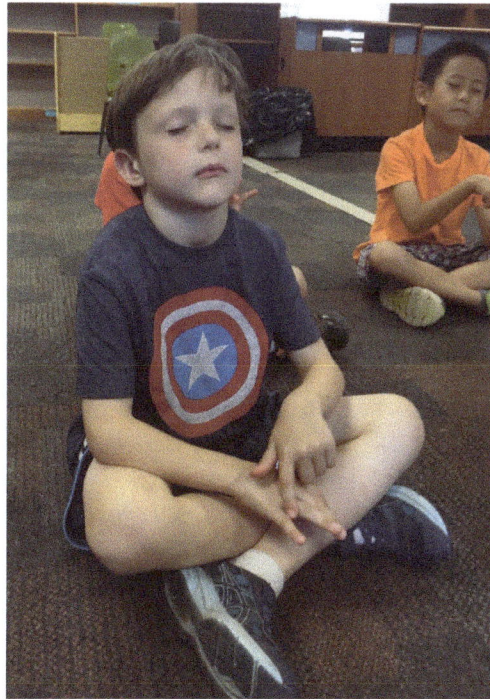

Week 7
Heartfulness

MINDFULNESS PRACTICE: Heartfulness

OBJECTIVES: Use the practice of thinking kind thoughts to increase feelings of compassion and empathy for yourself and others.

Practice kindness.

PREPARE: A bell or chime

Marleigh is Mindful

Your Kindness Pals list

Copies of Heartfulness Worksheet (in Resource Section)

Optional: Talking Object

Today we will introduce the compassion practice of Heartfulness. Heartfulness is a wonderful practice that can create a beautiful moment in your class. In this practice, students will think kind thoughts about themselves, someone they know, and the whole world.

> NOTE FROM LINDA: *You might want to steer their choices about who to think their kind thoughts about to people or animals that they see every day. Otherwise a lot of kids tend to think of people or pets who have died. I've seen this happen a lot. Of course there is nothing wrong with thinking about or talking about those we have loved and lost, but it can become very upsetting for some kids and might be triggering for those who have experienced a profound loss, and you may not have the resources to respond as you would want to in the moment. Do your best to give examples that keep the focus on someone they talk to every day or even a beloved stuffed animal.*

Mindfulness Practice

1. **Introduce Heartfulness.**

   Say: *Today we are going to do something called Heartfulness. This just means that we are going to be thinking about a person and sending them kind thoughts.*

   We aren't going to be making them a card or talking to them. We are going to be thinking kind thoughts about them in our minds. Let's start out as we always do with our Mindfulness Helper and then I'll let you know what we are going to do.

   Invite today's Mindfulness Helper (MH) to come to the front of the class to sit next to you on a chair (or next to you on the floor).

   Say: *Let's all be happy for* _____. *(sign language applause)*

   Say: *Today we are going to practice our Take 5 breathing with our eyes closed.*

   Prompt the MH to say: "Let's get into our mindful bodies. Let's close our eyes or look down. Let's take three deep breaths."

   Check to see that all students are sitting comfortably with their eyes closed or looking down keeping in mind that for some children this will be difficult. Keep your expectations reasonable given what you know about your students.

   Say: *I'd like you to think about someone who makes you happy.* **Choose someone you see every day** *at home or at school. You might choose someone in your family, a friend, teacher, even a pet. Just choose someone and try to picture that person happy and smiling. Picture them doing something that makes them happy. Try to notice how you feel when you think about this person.*

   Now, if you'd like to, fill your heart up with kindness and repeat these words in your mind while you think about this person. I will say the words out loud and you may think them in your mind or whisper them quietly.

   May you be happy. **Wait a moment to give them time to repeat the words.**

   May you be healthy. **Wait a moment.**

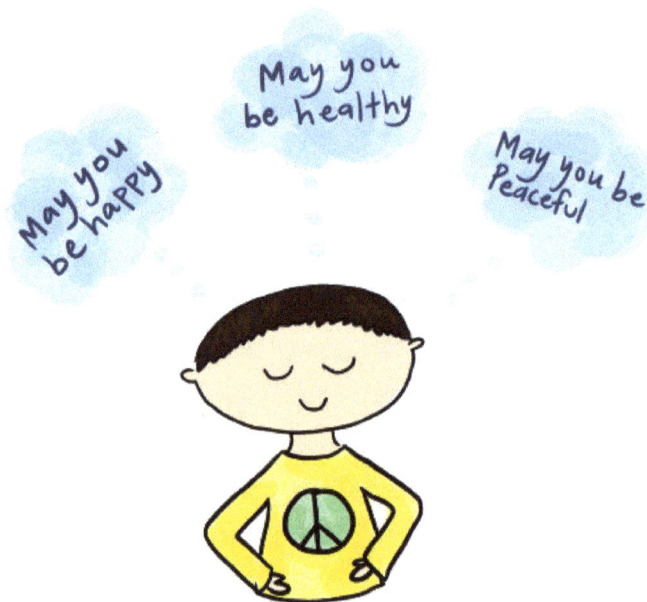

May you be peaceful. **Wait a moment.**

Take a moment to notice how you feel. Any way that you feel is fine, even if you feel nothing. Just try to notice it.

Now take a deep breath, and listen for the sound of the bell. Try to listen to the whole sound of the bell. Open your eyes or look up when you cannot hear it anymore.

Ask the MH to ring the bell when the mindful breathing is complete.

Ask the MH to return to their seat.

Invite the students to share whom they were thinking about or how it felt.

Read and Discuss

Marleigh is Mindful

Say: *Today let's see who uses Heartfulness in Marleigh is Mindful. It's Sophie! Let's hear about Sophie's experience.*

Read the two pages on Sophie and Heartfulness Breathing.

Ask:

Why did Sophie practice Heartfulness?

How could Heartfulness help you?

Activity: Heartfulness worksheet

Say: *Now we are going to draw a picture of the person or animal you were thinking about during Heartfulness.*

Hand out the Heartfulness worksheet and give the children time to draw a picture. If you have time you can have them share their pictures with the class or with their Kindness Pals.

Kindness Pals

Do the Kindness Pals activity as before.

Closing Words: *Let's have a nice quiet moment with the bell. You can close your eyes or leave them open, but let's sit quietly and listen to the bell. If you want to, you can think about your new Kindness Pal and imagine yourself doing something kind for him or her.*

Ring the bell or chime. *Thanks for a great class, everyone.*

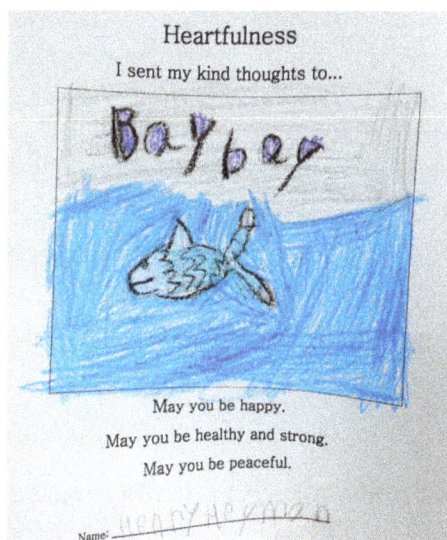

Moving Mindfully

MINDFULNESS PRACTICE: Candle Breaths

OBJECTIVES:
Learn how Mindful Movements help to connect our bodies and minds and heighten our sense of control over our bodies.

Practice Candle Breaths.

Practice kindness.

PREPARE:
A bell or chime

Marleigh is Mindful by Linda Ryden

Music for Freeze Dancing. You can use music that is calm and encourages peaceful movement or you can use music that changes tempo and mood frequently.

Your Kindness Pal list

Optional:
Talking Object

This week we explore a new Mindful Breathing Practice called Candle Breaths, another way to help children calm themselves down. We are learning many quiet mindfulness practices in this unit, including mindful breathing, mindful seeing and mindful listening. But as we've mentioned before, mindfulness practice does not have to be still or quiet. We can also self-regulate using movement. Mindful movement can help connect our minds with our bodies and help us develop a sense of control over our actions, even in the middle of big emotions. This week we introduce Mindful Movement through the Mirror Game and Freeze Dancing. Have fun!

Mindfulness Practice

1. **Practice mindful breathing with Candle Breaths**

   Invite today's Mindfulness Helper (MH) to come to the front of the class to sit next to you on a chair (or next to you on the floor).

   Say: *Let's all be happy for _____.* (sign language applause)

Say: *Today we are going to try something called Candle Breaths. Imagine your favorite birthday cake - imagine the flavors, the decorations, everything about it. Now imagine that it is time to blow out the birthday candles. Breathe in gently and when you breathe out, imagine that you are blowing out your birthday candles. Happy birthday!*

Prompt the MH to say: "Let's get into our mindful bodies. Let's close our eyes or look down. Let's take three deep Candle Breaths."

Read and Discuss

Marleigh is Mindful

Say: *Today let's see who uses Candle Breathing in* Marleigh is Mindful. *It's Zivana! Let's hear about Zivana's experience.*

Read the two pages on Zivana and Persida and Candle Breathing.

Ask:

- How did Candle Breathing help Zivana?
- How could Candle Breathing help you?

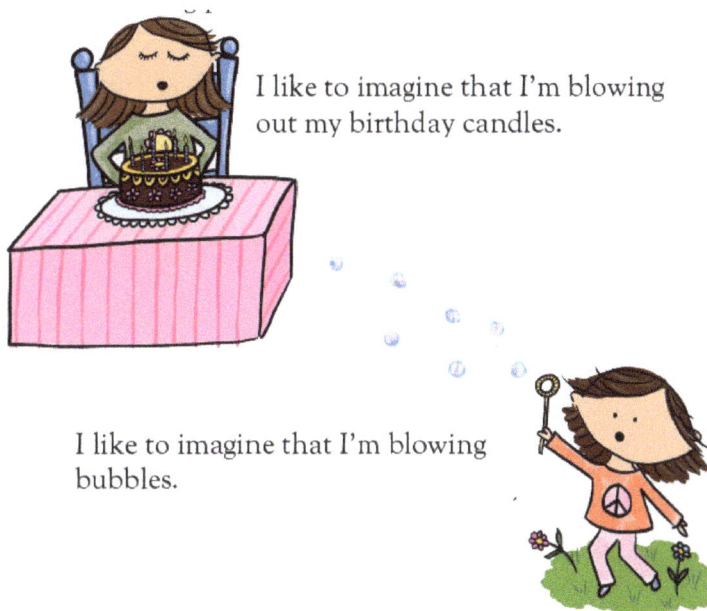

I like to imagine that I'm blowing out my birthday candles.

I like to imagine that I'm blowing bubbles.

Activity: The Mirror Game

Say: *Today we are going to be moving mindfully. What do you think it means to move mindfully?* Let some children share.

Instruct the children to stand up somewhere in the room where they will have a little bubble of space around them. Ask them to be mindful of other people's bodies when they choose their space. Use this as an opportunity to model moving mindfully.

Ask the children to pretend they are your reflections in the mirror and to keep their eyes on you the whole time.

Encourage the children to focus on what their bodies feel like when they are moving.

You might say: *Notice how heavy your arms feel when you hold them out in front of you.*

Vary the tempo of the movements to keep the children "on their toes."

Try doing movements very slowly to notice how many parts of the body are involved. Then do the movements quickly.

> *NOTE: Another fun variation is to play a form of "Simon Says," but don't let the kids get "out."*

Discuss

You might say: Let's take a few minutes to talk about how mindfulness practices like Candle Breathing can help to connect our bodies and minds.

Ask: When you are playing sports, or dancing, or playing an instrument, how could mindfulness help you control your movements?

Point out that when we can calm down, we are more able to move in the way we want to move. Instead of hitting another person when you are angry, you could use Candle Breaths to calm down so you could express your anger in another way.

Perhaps mention that some athletes use mindfulness to get ready for big games, especially when they are anxious, to help them calm down so they can think more clearly and move more easily than if they were worried or nervous.

Activity: Freeze Dancing

Say: *Now we are going to try another way of moving mindfully. We are going to play a game called Freeze Dance.*

I'm going to put on some music. When the music starts you can start to move your body in any way that feels good to you as long as you are being mindful of the other people around you.

We are not going to be making any noises because we are going to be busy listening and moving our bodies.

You have to listen carefully in Freeze Dancing because I am going to be turning the music on and off. When I turn the music off, you freeze. When I turn the music back on, you can unfreeze and start moving along with the music again.

No one will get "out." If you don't freeze, I'll ask you to try again. Ready? Let's go!

Play the game for a few minutes as long as it doesn't get out of control. You might remind some children about being mindful of other people's bodies and to really try to listen to the music.

Remember to try and put the guidelines in positive language such as, "As long as you follow the directions you can continue to play the game." This can be much more effective than the more traditional way of saying, "If you don't follow the rules you can't play." Many children react defiantly to orders like that but are perfectly happy to follow the rules when they are stated in a more neutral way.

Discuss

Talk about what it felt like to move mindfully.

Ask how moving mindfully could be important in school, e.g. walking through crowded hallways, navigating the cafeteria, and so on.

Do the Kindness Pals activity as before.

Closing Words: *Let's have a nice quiet moment with the bell. You can close your eyes or leave them open, but let's sit quietly and listen to the bell. If you want to, you can think about your new Kindness Pal and imagine yourself doing something kind for him or her.*

Ring the bell or chime. *Thanks for a great class, everyone.*

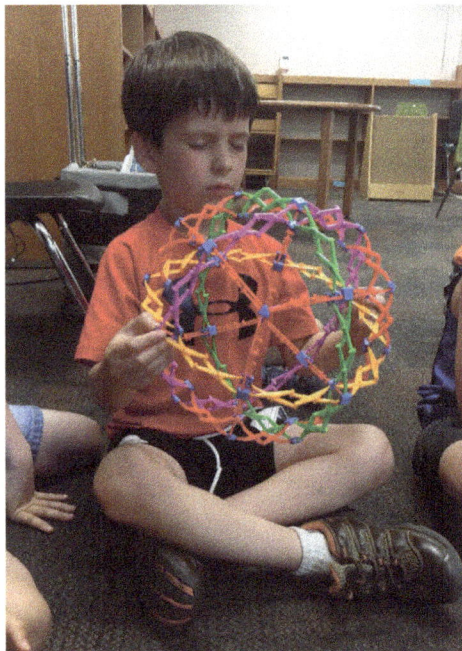

Wave Breathing

MINDFULNESS PRACTICE: Wave Breathing

Objectives:
- Experiment with deep breathing.
- Practice Wave Breathing.
- Practice kindness.

PREPARE:
- A bell or chime
- *Marleigh is Mindful* by Linda Ryden
- Your Kindness Pals list
- "Create Your Own Way of Breathing" Worksheet
- Optional: Talking Object

This week, we are introducing a new Mindful Breathing practice called Wave Breathing - one more for your students to try out and add to their collection. We are also inviting students to create their own breathing practices once again to help them develop a sense of ownership of their own practice and to help them focus on their own personal experiences and benefits. This lesson has a slightly different rhythm as children will be developing their own practices first and practicing mindfulness with the Mindfulness Helper after that.

Mindfulness Practice

1. Introduce Wave Breathing

You might say:

Today I'm going to teach you a new way of breathing. It's called Wave breathing. Can anybody show the motion of a wave with your arms? Can you do it with your whole body?

We're going to do a similar movement while we do our deep breathing. Let me show you.

Demonstrate: Breathe in while you lift your arms in an upward wave-like motion and then breathe out as you bring your arm down like "the wave" that people do at sports events. Do this a few times.

Now let's try it together. Let's get into our mindful bodies. Let's take three deep wave breaths.

2. **Create your own way of deep breathing.**

Say: *Great! Now let's think of more ways to do our deep breathing. Do you remember a few weeks ago we did Animal Breathing? Let's try that again, only this time let's think of other things in nature like the wind, or water, and let's breathe like them.*

Demonstrate your own way of breathing, and ask the children to follow you.

Say: *Can you think of some other ways that we could breathe?*

Let everyone have a chance to demonstrate their ideas, and let everyone try each creation once or twice. Remind the children that the movement should be slow and peaceful to go along with the gentle feeling of deep breathing. Some ideas might be waterfall breathing, rainbow breathing, wind breathing, etc.

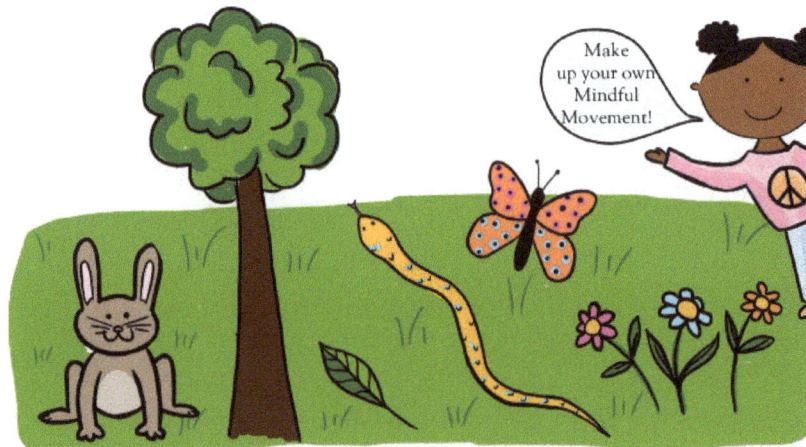

3. Practice your own way of deep breathing.

Invite today's Mindfulness Helper (MH) to come to the front of the class to sit next to you on a chair (or next to you on the floor).

Say: *Let's all be happy for _____.* *(sign language applause)*

Say: *The Mindfulness Helper is going to get us set up. When s/he says "Let's take three deep breaths…," you can do your breaths any way that you want to. You can do the breathing that you just created, or you can do someone else's. Just make sure that your breaths are slow and quiet.*

Prompt the MH to say: "Let's get into our mindful bodies. Let's close our eyes or look down. Let's take three deep breaths."

Now listen for the sound of the bell. Try to listen to the whole sound of the bell. Open your eyes or look up when you cannot hear it anymore.

Ask the MH to ring the bell when the mindful breathing is complete.

Ask the MH to return to their seat.

Read and Discuss

Marleigh is Mindful

Say: *Today let's see who makes up their own mindfulness breathing practices in Marleigh is Mindful. It's Angelo! Let's hear about Angelo's experience.*

Read the two pages on Angelo and the practices that he makes up.

Ask*:*

- Why did Angelo make up his own Mindful Movements?
- Which one of Angelo's movements would you like to use?

Activity: Drawing

To help children remember the practices they have created, and to make it easier to share them at home, pass out the "Create Your Own Way of Breathing" worksheet.

Invite the students to draw a picture of their new way of breathing.

Kindness Pals

Do the Kindness Pal activity as before.

Closing Words: *Let's have a nice quiet moment with the bell. You can close your eyes or leave them open, but let's sit quietly and listen to the bell. If you want to, you can think about your new Kindness Pal and imagine yourself doing something kind for him or her.*

Ring the bell or chime. *Thanks for a great class, everyone.*

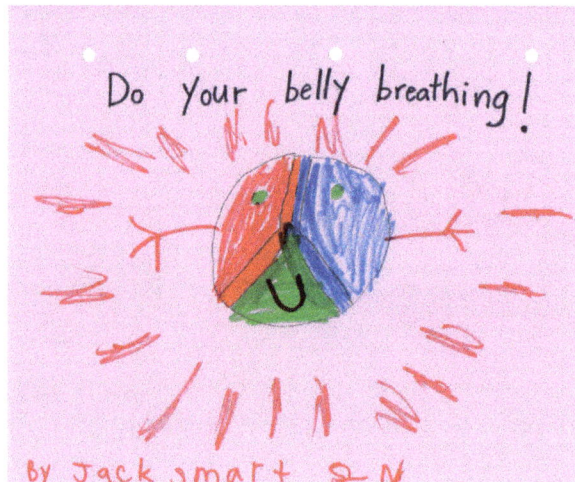

UNIT 2:
Gratitude

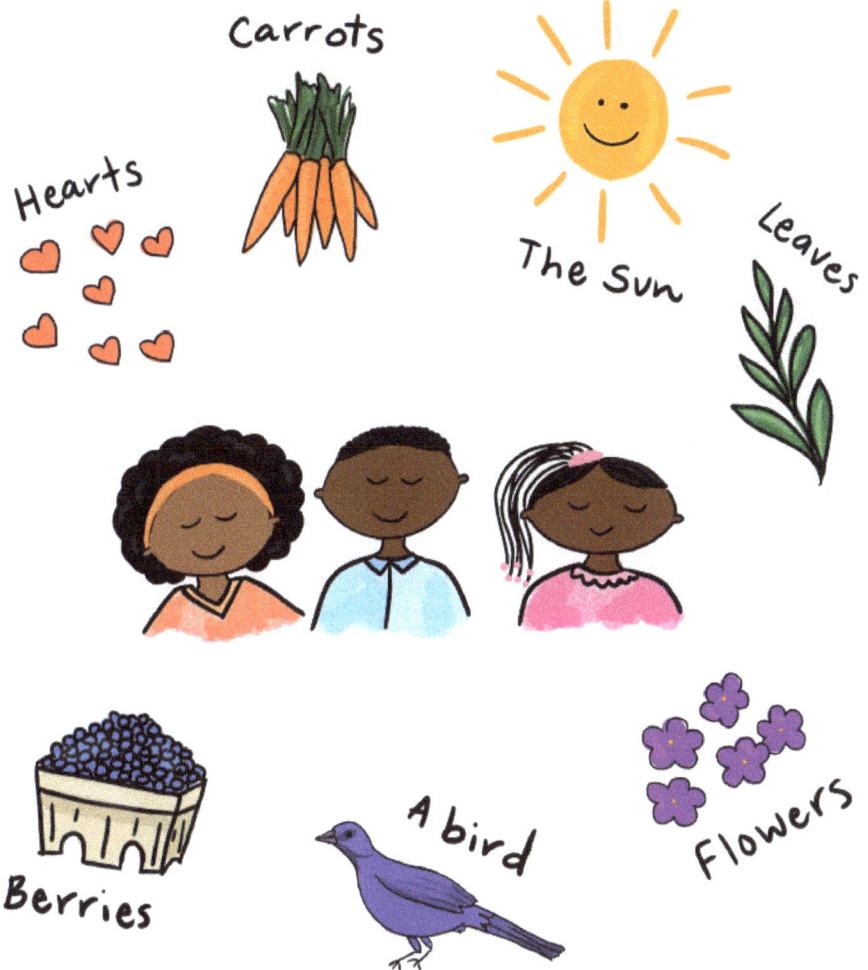

Carrots

Hearts

The Sun

Leaves

Berries

A bird

Flowers

Week 10
Feeling Grateful

MINDFULNESS PRACTICE: Gravity Hands

OBJECTIVES: Learn how to develop a gratitude practice.

Introduce Gravity Hands.

Practice kindness.

PREPARE: A bell or chime

Your Kindness Pals list

Marleigh is Mindful by Linda Ryden

Listen to the refrain of the song "Tell Me Something Good" by Chaka Kahn. This is for YOU, not the students!

Copies of the "I am grateful for…" worksheet

Optional: Talking Object

The purpose of this lesson is to help children develop the habit of gratitude and of noticing the little good things in life. Our brains are wired to look for trouble and to really focus on it, allowing us to learn from negative experiences so that we don't repeat them. Gratitude practice helps us balance this tendency.

This lesson uses an old song in a new way. **Don't play the song for your class.** *Instead, listen to the song "Tell Me Something Good" by Chaka Khan as you prepare the lesson. The only part you'll be using with your class is the refrain "Tell me something good."* **The rest of the song is not appropriate for school,** *although the kids might have heard parts of it in TV commercials. If you are not comfortable singing, you can just say the words. Or make up your own song or chant. Have fun with it!*

Mindfulness Practice

1. Introduce Gravity Hands

Gravity Hands is a very simple practice of slowly moving your hands up when you breathe in and then slowly lowering them down when you breathe out. It's fun to think about gravity while doing this practice. Making your inhale and exhale the same length can be very soothing and calming.

Say: *Today we're going to learn another way of doing mindful breathing called Gravity Hands! Start out by stretching your arms straight out in front of you with your palms facing down. Hold them there and I'm going to count 30 seconds. (wait 30 seconds) So what are you noticing? Are your arms starting to feel heavy, do you want to put them down? Is it getting harder? Let's put our arms down now.*

Ask: *Does anybody know why our arms started to feel heavy or it was hard to hold them up? It's because of gravity! Gravity is a force that pulls things down toward the earth. It's the reason that we aren't floating around the classroom right now! When we throw a ball up in the air what happens to it? That's right, it falls back down.*

You can have kids demonstrate gravity by jumping up and noticing that they come right back down or dropping a feather and watching it fall.

Say: *Gravity is why it was hard to keep our arms outstretched - gravity wanted them to come down. Let's try it again.*

Repeat the arm activity from above reminding them to notice the pull of gravity.

Say: *Today we're going to do a mindful breathing practice called Gravity Hands. We're going to slowly bring our hands up, palms up, and then we're going to turn them over and slowly bring them down, palms down. Let's try that a few times,*

Now we're going to add breathing to it. When we slowly bring our hands up we're going to breathe in slowly and gently. When we lower our hands back down we're going to breathe out slowly and gently.

Let's try it for our Mindful Moment!

2. **Practice Mindfulness with the Mindfulness Helper**

Invite today's Mindfulness Helper (MH) to come to the front of the class to sit next to you on a chair (or next to you on the floor).

Say: *Let's all be happy for* _____. *(sign language applause)*

Prompt the MH to say: "Let's get into our mindful bodies. Let's close our eyes or look down. Let's do Gravity Hands."

You or the Mindfulness Helper can lead the class through the practice again.

Ask the MH to ring the bell when the mindful breathing is complete.

Ask the MH to return to their seat.

Read and Discuss

Marleigh is Mindful

Say: *Today let's see who practices Gravity Hands in* Marleigh is Mindful. *It's Navaneet! Let's hear about Navaneet's experience.*

Read the two pages on Navaneet and why he practices Gravity Hands.

Ask:

- How did Gravity Hands help Navaneet?
- How could Gravity Hands be helpful to you?

Gratitude Practice

1. Introduce the concept of gratitude.

Say: *Today we are going to be talking about gratitude. Does anybody want to guess what that word means? Gratitude means being thankful or grateful. When we are grateful, or feeling gratitude, we notice good things or people, and we feel thankful for them.*

Maybe you feel grateful because it is sunny out today. Or maybe you are grateful because it is raining and your garden will grow. Maybe you are grateful that your shoes are comfortable and not tight. Maybe you are filled with gratitude because it is almost time for recess.

2. Introduce gratitude practice and the song.

Say: *Sometimes it can be easy to forget to notice these little good things in life, so we are going to practice being grateful and mindfully noticing. And to make it even more fun, we are going to sing a little song about it.*

I'm going to ask you to think of a little good thing in your life and raise your hand. When I call on you we'll all sing "tell me something good" and then you will. I'll go first. Sing it with me, "tell me something good"! And I'll tell you that I had waffles for breakfast or [Insert your own answer here]. Now it's your turn.

Call on whomever raises their hand and **say or sing**: "[Child's Name], tell me something good…"

Try to leave enough time for everyone to share. If the kids start to head in the direction of getting things like video games, or vacations, remind them to focus on the little good things.

This is a practice that you will be repeating in subsequent lessons. You might want to vary it by asking them to share good things they noticed in nature, or kind things that they did for others or that others did for them, or good things they had to eat recently.

Be creative and have fun with it. Students really love this. If you don't feel comfortable singing - feel free to just use it as a prompt or a chant or make up your own way of doing it!

Activity: I am grateful for...

Hand out copies of the "I am grateful for…" worksheet.

Say: *Now we're going to draw a picture of something that you are grateful for. It can be a person who makes you happy, a pet, your teddy bear, or your lunch. Anything is fine.*

If you have time let the children share their drawings with the class or perhaps with their Kindness Pals.

Kindness Pals

Do the Kindness Pals activity as before.

Closing Words: *Let's have a nice quiet moment with the bell. You can close your eyes or leave them open, but let's sit quietly and listen to the bell. If you want to, you can think about your new Kindness Pal and imagine yourself doing something kind for him or her.*

Ring the bell or chime. *Thanks for a great class, everyone.*

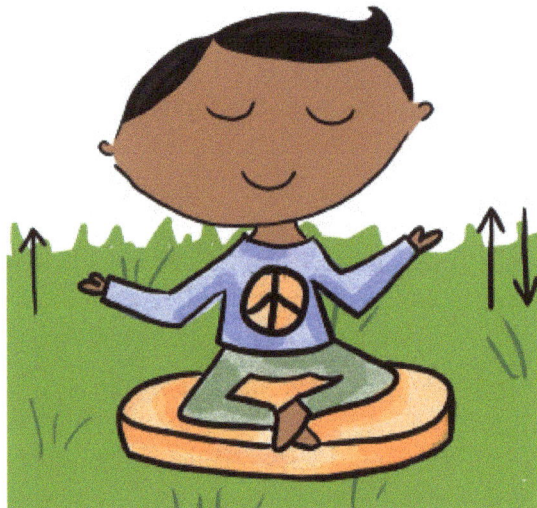

Week 11
Sergio Sees the Good

MINDFULNESS PRACTICE: Cup of Gratitude

OBJECTIVES: Learn about the Negativity Bias and how we can help our brains remember little good things.

Practice kindness.

PREPARE: A bell or chime

Sergio Sees the Good by Linda Ryden

Your Kindness Pals list

Optional: Talking Object

This week we will be talking about a powerful concept: how gratitude practice can balance out our brain's tendency to focus on negative things, called the negativity bias. Bad things do happen, and often we let them overshadow all of the small good things that also fill our days. By using the gratitude practices in this lesson, we can balance out our perception of our days which can make us feel happier.

Introduction

Say: *Do you remember last time when we talked about gratitude? Does anybody remember what that word means? That's right - It means being grateful or thankful. We practiced being grateful for the little good things in our lives. Today we're going to learn another way to practice gratitude and we're going to read a new book called* Sergio Sees the Good.

Today we're going to be making a Cup of Gratitude. We'll be thinking about people or things that we are grateful for and we'll be imagining that we are putting them in our little cup. Can you make a little cup with your hands? Imagine you are going to drink some water and use your hands as a cup - can you do that? Now we're going to be thinking about people, animals, and things that we are grateful or thankful for. We're going to imagine that they are really tiny and can fit into our cupped hands. Let's get started.

Mindfulness Practice

Invite today's Mindfulness Helper (MH) to come to the front of the class to sit next to you on a chair.

Prompt the MH to say: *"Let's get into our mindful bodies; Let's close our eyes or look down; Let's take three deep breaths."*

Say: *So let's begin:*

Let's start by making our gratitude cups with our hands.

Now try to think about someone at home that you see every day or almost every day that you are thankful, or grateful for. Think of someone who helps you and is kind to you. Now imagine that you can hold them in your little Cup of Gratitude.

Now let's take a deep breath in and as you breathe out, whisper "thank you" into your little cup.

Maybe there is a special animal in your life such as a pet or a stuffed animal or an animal in the wild. Imagine that they are in your little Cup of Gratitude. Let's send some thanks to that animal. Take a deep breath in and as you breathe out, whisper "thank you" into your little cup.

Next, let's think about someone in your class who is kind to you. Imagine that they are in your little Cup of Gratitude. Let's send some thanks to that person. Take a deep breath in and as you breathe out, whisper "thank you" into your little cup.

Take a moment to soak in this feeling of gratitude. Notice what it feels like to be grateful and to say thank you. Remember that you can do this practice on your own anytime.

Let's take a deep breath in and stretch your arms up over your head and then slowly float your arms down as you breathe out. Let's listen for the sound of the bell and we'll open our eyes or look up when we can't hear it anymore.

Say: *In a moment you will hear the sound of the bells and that will mean that it is time to open your eyes or look up. So just get ready for that.*

Ask the MH to ring the bell and return to their seat.

Read and Discuss: The Negativity Bias and *Sergio Sees the Good*

Say: *Today we're going to read a book called* Sergio Sees the Good. *This is a book that teaches us about why it's so important to notice the little good things in life. We'll also learn something new about our brains!*

Read *Sergio Sees the Good*

As Sergio's mom adds marbles to their scale, have kids keep track of how many marbles are on each side of the scale. You can ask them to make tally marks on a piece of paper or a white board, or do it on their fingers or in their minds.

Ask:

Did Sergio really have a completely terrible day?

What are the little good things that he forgot all about?

Why do you think Sergio only remembered that one bad thing?

Activity:

Now we're going to sit with our new Kindness Pal and you can each share one good thing and one bad thing that happened to you today.

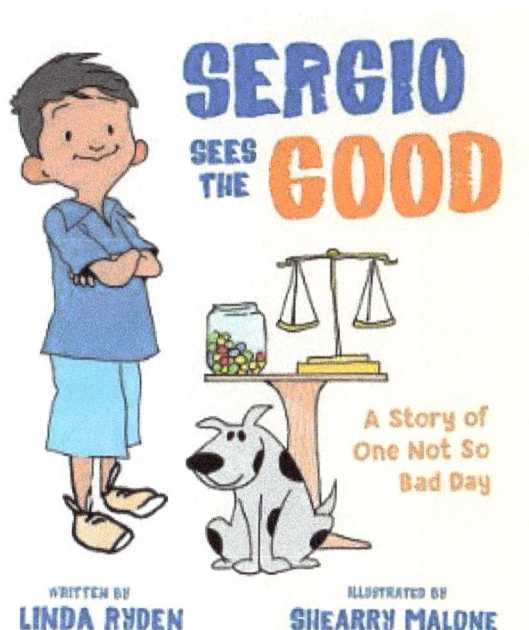

SERGIO SEES THE GOOD

A Story of One Not So Bad Day

WRITTEN BY LINDA RYDEN   ILLUSTRATED BY SHEARRY MALONE

Kindness Pals

Do the Kindness Pals activity as before.

Closing Words: *Let's have a nice quiet moment with the bell. You can close your eyes or leave them open, but let's sit quietly and listen to the bell. If you want to, you can think about your new Kindness Pal and imagine yourself doing something kind for him or her.*

Ring the bell or chime. *Thanks for a great class, everyone.*

Gratitude Marble Game

MINDFULNESS PRACTICE:	Choose: Take 5, Wave Breathing, Gravity Hands.
	Gratitude practice.
OBJECTIVES:	Practice training our brains to notice little good things.
	Reinforce lessons about the Negativity Bias.
	Practice kindness.
PREPARE:	A bell or chime
	Your Kindness Pals list
	Little cups (one for each student) and marbles or pasta, paperclips, any small things that you have a lot of (five or so for each student)
	Optional: Talking Object

Today we are going to continue learning about the impact of noticing the little good things. Noticing the little good things can help our brains not to just focus on bad things that happen. We're not trying to sweep bad things under the rug or ignore them - but we are trying to make sure that our brains don't convince us that things are worse than they really are.

In our mindfulness practices, we invite kids to choose among 3 practices they have learned for today's practice.

Mindfulness Practice

1. Gratitude Practice: Tell me Something Good

Say: *Sometimes it can be easy to forget to notice these little good things in life, so we are going to practice being grateful and mindfully noticing. And to make it even more fun, we are going to sing a little song about it. Do you remember when we did this a couple of weeks ago?*

I'm going to ask you to think of a little good thing in your life and then raise your hand. When I call on you, we'll all sing "tell me something good" and then you will tell us your good thing. I'll go first. Sing it with me, "tell me something good"! And I'll tell you that I had waffles for breakfast or [Insert your own answer here]. Now it's your turn.

Call on whomever raises their hand and **say or sing**: "[Child's Name], tell me something good…" Try to leave enough time for everyone to share. If the kids start to head in the direction of getting things like video games, or vacations, remind them to focus on the little good things.

2. **Vote on a Mindfulness Practice**

   Before you begin, ask the class what kind of breathing they would like to practice today. Let them choose between Take Five Breathing, Wave Breathing, or Gravity Hands. Take a vote. This can be a fun way to keep them excited about the practice.

   Invite today's Mindfulness Helper (MH) to come to the front of the class to sit next to you on a chair (or next to you on the floor).

   Say: *Let's all be happy for _____.* (sign language applause)

   Prompt the MH to say: "Let's get into our mindful bodies. Let's close our eyes or look down. Let's (insert whatever they decided to do here.)"

   Say: *Now let your breath settle back into its natural rhythm. Just breathe. Put your hand on your belly and try to make your body so still and quiet that the only thing that you can feel moving is your breath.*

   Wait a few moments to see how long they can hold this focus.

   Say: *Now take a deep breath, and listen for the sound of the bell. Try to listen to the whole sound of the bell. Open your eyes when you cannot hear it anymore.*

   Ask the MH to ring the bell and return to their seat.

Activity: Gratitude Marble Game:

> NOTE FROM LINDA: *This is one of the most popular activities in my classroom! If you have time you can do this several times throughout the school year.*

In this activity, you will help the children try to remember all of the little good things that happened to Sergio. If you have a balance scale you can use that for this, otherwise just use two cups and some marbles or whatever little objects you have around.

Say: *Today we are going to play a game that will help us to train our brains to notice the little good things. Do you remember in Sergio Sees the Good his mother got out a scale and some marbles and they tried to remember everything that happened to Sergio that day?*

We're going to try to remember all of the good and bad things that happened to Sergio and we're going to put a marble in the good side (or cup) for all the good things and a marble in the bad side (or cup) for all the bad things.

Go through the story with the class and see if they can remember what happened.

Say: *Do you remember that Sergio told his mom that he had a totally terrible day? Was he right? That's right - he had forgotten about most of the good things that happened. His brain was really focused on the one bad thing that happened and that was all that he was remembering.*

Instruct: *Now you're going to get a chance to try it! First I'm going to tell you who your new Kindness Pal is. Then I'm going to give you and your Kindness Pal two cups and some marbles (or pasta, paperclips, whatever you have). You are going to sit across from each other with the cups in between you. You can choose one cup to be the Good cup and one cup to be the Bad cup.*

Then you are going to decide who goes first. That person will be the talker and the other person will hold the marbles. The talker will try to remember everything that happened yesterday and the marble holder will put marbles in the good cup for good things and in the bad cup for bad things. At the end you can count how many marbles are in each cup. Then you will switch places. Try to remember lots of little details.

Give them about 5-10 minutes for this. It's a powerful practice because not only are they thinking about and remembering little good things but they are really listening to each other and witnessing each other's lives.

When the time is up ask the kids to reflect on how many good and bad marbles they had in each cup and what it felt like to do the activity

Kindness Pals

Do the Kindness Pals activity as before.

Closing Words: *Let's have a nice quiet moment with the bell. You can close your eyes or leave them open, but let's sit quietly and listen to the bell. If you want to, you can think about your new Kindness Pal and imagine yourself doing something kind for him or her.*

Ring the bell or chime. *Thanks for a great class, everyone.*

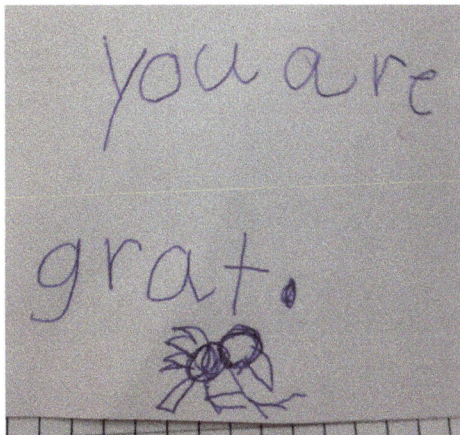

Week 13
Gratefuls Box

MINDFULNESS PRACTICE: Straw Breathing

OBJECTIVES: Practice gratitude by making a Gratefuls Box.

Learn about hacking the Negativity Bias with gratitude.

Practice kindness.

PREPARE: A bell or chime

Your Kindness Pals list

For this activity you can use brown paper bags, clear baggies, empty tissue boxes, whatever you have around. You just need enough for everyone in your class.

Little strips of paper - about 2 inches long

Another option is to use the Gratefuls Box Worksheet (see Worksheet Section)

Optional: Talking Object

Today we are going to continue learning about the impact of noticing the little good things and expressing gratitude for them. Gratitude practice has been shown to have many benefits such as increasing our sense of well-being and decreasing stress. You can encourage students to use this practice, like all of the others taught here, at home as well as at school. A video of Linda Ryden reading Sergio Sees the Good is available at no charge on the Peace of Mind website, TeachPeaceofMind.org. Feel free to share the link with your families!

Mindfulness Practice

1. Gratitude Practice: Tell me Something Good

Say: *Sometimes it can be easy to forget to notice these little good things in life, so we are going to practice being grateful and mindfully noticing. And to make it even more fun, we are going to sing a little song about it. Do you remember when we did this a couple of weeks ago?*

I'm going to ask you to think of a little good thing in your life and then raise your hand. When I call on you, we'll all sing "tell me something good" and then you will tell us your good thing. I'll go first. Sing it with me, "tell me something good"! And I'll tell you that I had waffles for breakfast or [Insert your own answer here]. Now it's your turn.

Call on whomever raises their hand and **say or sing**: "[Child's Name], tell me something good…" Try to leave enough time for everyone to share. If the kids start to head in the direction of getting things like video games, or vacations, remind them to focus on the little good things.

2. **Straw Breathing**

Straw Breathing can be a helpful practice to help kids to calm down when they are feeling anxious or nervous. It involves a gentle inhale and then a long, slow, controlled exhale. This combination has been shown to be effective in helping to calm the amygdala - the brain's security guard. When the amygdala senses danger it puts us into a fight, flight, or freeze mode. Most of the time in those states we start breathing in a faster, more shallow way. Deliberately slowing down the exhale and paying attention to it can help send a message to our amygdala that we are not in immediate danger. We'll be learning about the amygdala in Week 21.

Introduce the practice: *Today we're going to learn a new way of doing Mindful Breathing. So far we have learned Animal Breaths, Tummy Breaths, Take Five Breathing, Wave Breathing, Candle Breaths and we have created our own.*

Ask a student to demonstrate each breathing practice as you name them.

Say: *Today we're going to learn a new practice called Straw Breathing. We're going to pretend that we have a little, tiny straw - like you would have in a juice box. We're going to pretend to put the straw in our mouth, and breathe in through our nose, and then pretend that we are breathing out through the little straw. We're going to see how long we can make that out-breath or exhale last. I'll go first.*

Demonstrate and have the kids count how long you hold your exhale. Be sure to do it comfortably, we don't want to exaggerate the exhale to a point of discomfort.

Have the class try it a few times and share how it felt.

Say: *Another way to do Straw Breathing is to pretend that you are blowing bubbles into a drink. Do you ever do this? Let's try it.*

Give them time to try both ways of doing Straw Breathing.

Say: *Straw breathing can be a great way to help us to calm down when we feel nervous or worried.*

We have been learning a lot of different ways of doing mindful breathing so that you can choose the ones that you like best. We're all different and what works for me might not work for you and vice versa. We'll keep learning lots of different ways and you can try them out and see which ones work for you!

Let's try Straw Breathing now for our Mindful Moment.

3. **Mindful Moment**

    Invite today's Mindfulness Helper (MH) to come to the front of the class to sit next to you on a chair.

    Prompt the MH to say: *"Let's get into our mindful bodies; Let's close our eyes or look down; Let's take three deep breaths."*

    Say: *Let's take a deep breath in and stretch your arms up over your head and then slowly float your arms down as you breathe out. Let's listen for the sound of the bell and we'll open our eyes when we can't hear it anymore.*

    Say: *In a moment you will hear the sound of the bells and that will mean that it is time to open your eyes or look up. So just get ready for that.*

    Ask the MH to ring the bell.

    If needed, ask the MH to choose a classmate to turn the lights on.

    Ask the MH to return to their seat.

Activity: Gratefuls Box

Today students are going to make a "Gratefuls Box," a place to keep reminders of what they are grateful for. You can do this any way that you like. If you are into crafts you can have the kids decorate small boxes with stickers, drawing, feathers, whatever you've got. If you are using paper bags, you can have them decorate the bag. If you don't have supplies for this, you can have them draw a Gratefuls Box and then draw what they would put into it on the Gratefuls Box Worksheet.

Say: *Today we are going to make something to remember to look for and remember those little good things we've been talking about. We're going to make something called a Gratefuls Box (or bag).*

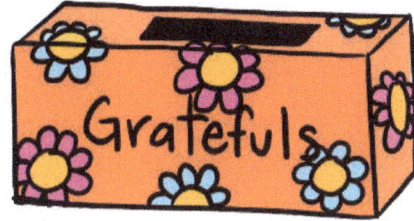

Say: *After you are done decorating your Gratefuls Box I'm going to pass out some strips of paper. You can write down or draw things you are grateful or thankful for on these little strips of paper and put them into your box. When you get home you can keep adding to your box. You might want to ask your family to join you. You could put the box in your kitchen and ask your family to add their own "Gratefuls" to the box.*

Read and Discuss

Marleigh is Mindful

Say: *Today let's see who has a Gratefuls Box in* Marleigh is Mindful. *It's Peyton! Let's hear about Peyton's experience.*

Read the two pages on Peyton and her Gratefuls box.

Ask*:*

- When Peyton feels sad or lonely, how does her Gratefuls box help her?
- What's one thing you will put in your Gratefuls box?

Kindness Pals

Do the Kindness Pals activity as before.

Closing Words: *Let's have a nice quiet moment with the bell. You can close your eyes or leave them open, but let's sit quietly and listen to the bell. If you want to, you can think about your new Kindness Pal and imagine yourself doing something kind for him or her.*

Ring the bell or chime. *Thanks for a great class, everyone.*

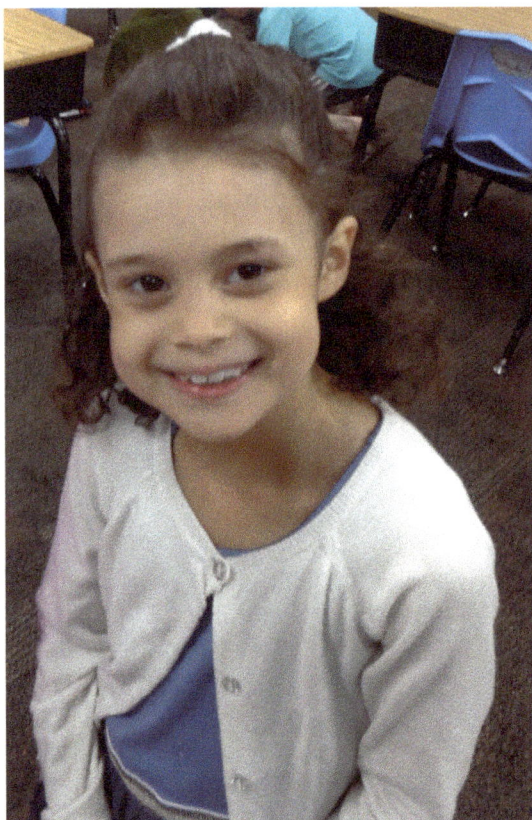

UNIT 3:
Feelings and Sensations

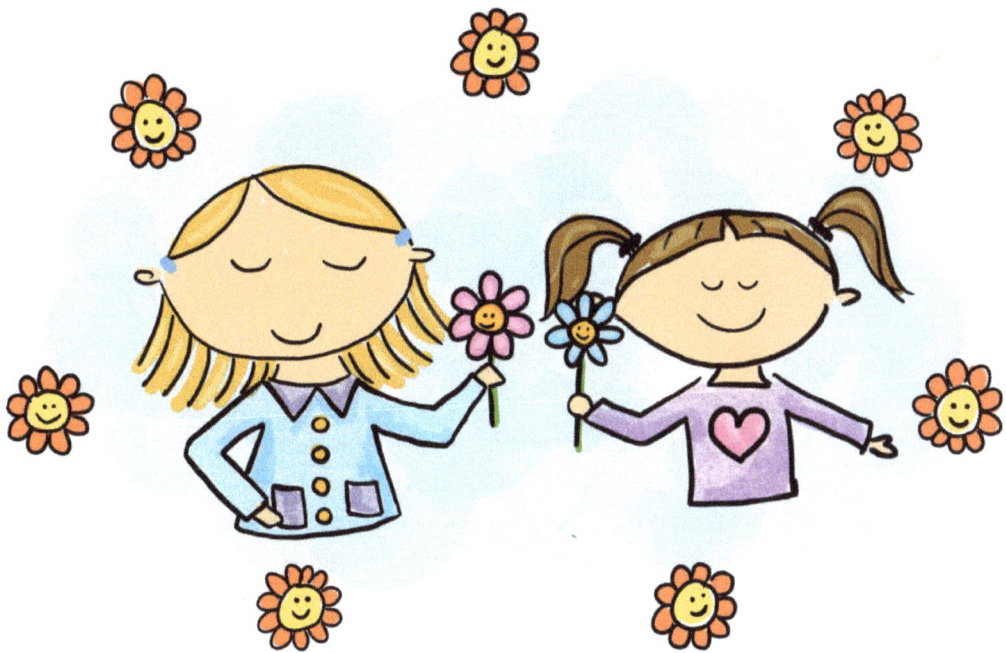

Week 14
Mindfulness of Sensations

MINDFULNESS PRACTICE: Noticing Sensations

OBJECTIVES::

Practice a new mindfulness exercise.

Learn that we can be aware of what is happening in our bodies.

Practice kindness.

PREPARE:

A bell or chime

Your Kindness Pals list

Kindness Pal Same and Different Worksheet

Optional: Talking Object

Today we will explore sensations - physical experiences in our bodies. Becoming more aware of physical sensations can help us to notice when we are beginning to experience a big emotion so that we can take care of it before it overwhelms us. We will start with the gratitude practice "Tell Me Something Good" again this week.

Gratitude Practice

Repeat the "Tell me something good" lesson from last week.

Say: *I'm going to ask you to think of a little good thing in your life and raise your hand. When I call on you, we'll all sing "tell me something good," and then you will. I'll go first. Sing it with me, "tell me something good"! And I'll tell you that I am happy because [Insert your own answer here]. Now it's your turn.*

Call on whomever raises their hand and **say or sing**: "[Child's Name], tell me something good..."

Try to leave enough time for everyone to share. Remind the kids to focus on the little good things.

Mindfulness Practice

1. **Introduce the word "sensation."**

   Say: *Today we're going to try something different. We're going to be focusing on our bodies and on different sensations. Does anybody want to guess what the word sensation means?*

   Give them time to guess.

   Say: *Sensations are physical feelings in your body. Have you ever had a mosquito bite? How does it feel? Well, that itchiness is a sensation.*

   Have you ever felt a breeze on your face? That feeling is a sensation. Today we're going to be focusing our minds on different sensations.

   First, I'm going to clap my hands and I want you to watch how I do it.

   Put your arms out in front of you with your palms facing each other, then clap your hands together hard. Leave your hands about a foot apart. You will notice an intense tingling feeling.

   Now I want you to close your eyes or look down into your lap if you don't feel comfortable closing your eyes, and put your arms out in front of you like I did. When I say 'Go' we are all going to clap our hands. Make sure that you don't talk, but just quietly notice what you feel. Go.

   Give them a moment to notice the sensation.

   Open your eyes when you can't feel that tingling anymore.

   Discuss what that felt like.

   Say: *Today we are going to take a little trip around our bodies with our minds and see if we can notice some sensations.*

2. **Practice mindfulness of sensations.**

   Invite today's Mindfulness Helper (MH) to come to the front of the class to sit next to you on a chair (or next to you on the floor).

   Say: *Let's all be happy for _____.* (sign language applause)

Prompt the MH to say: "Let's get into our mindful bodies. Let's close our eyes or look down. Let's take three deep Wave breaths."

Guide the class with these words:

Keeping your eyes closed, lift up one arm and put your hand in front of your mouth. Notice if it is hard to find your mouth with your eyes closed. Now gently blow on your hand. Notice what that feels like. Notice that sensation.

Now gently touch the top of your head. Notice what you feel in your hand. Notice what you feel in your head. Your hand is feeling your hair. Notice what that sensation feels like. Does your hand feel like a weight on your head?

Now put your hand out in front of you and wave it around gently. Do you feel air touching your hand? Does your arm feel tired? Notice what you feel.

Now put your hand on your knee. Notice the feeling of your skin or your clothes against your hand. What do you notice? Is the fabric of your clothing soft or scratchy? Does your skin feel warm or cool?

Now try to focus your mind on sensations in your feet. Choose one of your feet and wiggle your toes around a bit. See if you can move each one of your toes one at a time. Notice if one of your feet is warmer than the other.

Now let's take one more deep breath in and out. When you hear the sound of the breathing bell it will be time to open your eyes.

Ask the MH to ring the bell when the exercise is complete.

Ask the MH to return to their seat.

Discuss and reflect

Use these questions to guide a discussion.

- What did it feel like to focus on your body?
- What sensations did you notice?
- What did you notice when your hand was on the top of your head?
- What did you notice when your hand was on your knee?
- What did your feet feel like?
- Which one of your feet was the warmest?

Activity: Mirror Game

Say: *Remember when we played the Mirror Game a few weeks ago? When we played it then you all were trying to be my reflection in the mirror. This time you are going to work with your Kindness Pal and take turns being each other's reflection in the mirror.*

Assign the Kindness Pals as usual.

Instruct the children to stand up somewhere in the room where they will have a little bubble of space around them and stand face to face with their Kindness Pal. Ask them to be mindful of other people's bodies when they choose their space. Use this as an opportunity to model moving mindfully.

Ask the children to pretend they are their partner's reflection in the mirror and to keep their eyes on each other the whole time.

Encourage the children to focus on what their bodies feel like when they are moving.

You might say: *Notice how heavy your arms feel when you hold them out in front of you.*

Give them a minute or more for each person to have a turn being the leader.

Kindness Pals

Do the Kindness Pals activity as before.

Closing Words: *Let's have a nice quiet moment with the bell. You can close your eyes or leave them open, but let's sit quietly and listen to the bell. If you want to, you can think about your new Kindness Pal and imagine yourself doing something kind for him or her.*

Ring the bell or chime. *Thanks for a great class, everyone.*

Week 15
Mindful Eating

MINDFULNESS PRACTICE: Take Five, Mindful Eating

OBJECTIVES:
Practice mindful breathing and eating.

Apply our mindfulness skills to our everyday lives.

Practice kindness.

PREPARE:
A bell or chime

Enough raisins for all of your class to have one or two

Hand sanitizer

Your Kindness Pals list and Talking Object

Mindful eating is a practice that we introduce here with a raisin and that can be a powerful practice in general. Mindful eating helps us focus on the sensation of taste and using our five senses. We can eat mindfully as a self-care and compassion practice, too. Enjoy!

NOTE FROM LINDA: *Eating a raisin mindfully is a very common introductory mindfulness activity. I teach 500 children a week so I have to be very frugal when it comes to the mindful eating lesson, which is why I tend to stick with raisins. If your situation allows, be creative and add to this lesson by including orange slices or whole apples or another food that might be part of your students' culture. You might even combine this lesson with snack time if you are working with your own class. Just be mindful of allergens such as nuts and have fun!*

Mindfulness Practice

1. **Practice mindful breathing.**

   Invite today's Mindfulness Helper (MH) to come to the front of the class to sit next to you on a chair (or next to you on the floor).

   Say: *Let's all be happy for _____. (sign language applause)*

   Prompt the MH to say: "Let's get into our mindful bodies. Let's close our eyes or look down. Let's take three breaths."

   Say: *Now let's practice our Take Five breathing. Trace your hand while you breathe in and out five times.*

   Now take a deep breath, and listen for the sound of the bell. Try to listen to the whole sound of the bell. Open your eyes when you cannot hear it anymore.

   Ask the MH to ring the bell when the mindful breathing is complete.

   Ask the MH to return to their seat.

2. **Introduce and lead the Mindful Eating exercise.**

   Say: *Now we are going to see what it feels like to eat something mindfully.*

   Give everyone a raisin.

   You might say: *We are pretending to be scientists from another planet who have never seen this strange, shriveled up food object before. Our mission is to find out everything we can about it.*

   Ask the kids to hold the raisin in the palm of their hand.

   Mindfully observe.

   Say: *Okay, scientists. We are now going to explore this strange object. We will start out by using a very fancy piece of scientific equipment: the eyeball. Use your eyes to mindfully look at the raisin and see what you notice. Share with someone next to you what you notice and compare your observations.*

   Choose a few students to share what they noticed.

Mindfully touch.

Say: *Now we are going to use another fancy piece of scientific equipment: the index finger. With your index finger, just lightly touch the raisin and notice what you feel. Share your observations with someone next to you. Remember to be mindful of making sure that everyone has someone to share with.*

Choose a few students to share what they noticed.

Mindfully smell.

Say: *Now we are going to investigate this raisin with yet another fancy piece of scientific equipment* (see if they can guess what's next): *the nose. Carefully hold your raisin up to your nose and smell. What do you notice?*

Share your observations with someone next to you. Remember to be mindful of making sure that everyone has someone to share with.

Choose a few students to share what they noticed.

Mindfully listen.

Say: *Now I wonder what this raisin has to say? Hold your raisin between your thumb and index finger and put it up to your ear. Raise your hand if your raisin is talking. If not, try gently rolling the raisin back and forth and very mindfully listen to the sound it makes.*

What do you notice?

Share your observations with someone next to you. Remember to be mindful of making sure that everyone has someone to share with.

Choose a few students to share what they noticed.

Mindfully eat.

Say: *Now the time has finally come. It's time to taste the raisin.*

Give kids the option of skipping this part if they want to. Or encourage them to do as much as they can with the raisin with the freedom to spit it out or throw it away whenever they want to.

Remember, we are scientists, so we are not really concerned with whether or not we like the taste of the raisin. We are simply trying to learn about it. Let's start by investigating what it tastes like on different parts of our tongues. Start out by placing the raisin in the center of your tongue and notice what it tastes like, if anything. Then move it to the tip of your tongue, the sides, etc.

Now let's take one bite and then place the raisin back on your tongue. What do you notice? Is there a big difference between the taste of the outside of the raisin and the inside of the raisin? Give them time to answer. *Now slowly chew the rest of the raisin, noticing what you taste and then see how long you can feel the raisin after you swallow it.*

Then talk about how you can eat other foods mindfully.

In future classes, ask children if they tried mindful eating at home or school and what the experience was like.

Discuss and Reflect

Use these questions to help the class reflect on their experience.

- What did it feel like to eat mindfully?
- Is this the way you usually eat?
- Can you imagine yourself eating your dinner mindfully tonight?

Say*: Your assignment is to try to eat one thing mindfully today. Enjoy!*

Kindness Pals

Do the Kindness Pal activity as before.

If there is not enough time for sharing, you can skip that, but be sure to give the students new Kindness Pals.

Closing Words: *Let's have a nice quiet moment with the bell. You can close your eyes or leave them open, but let's sit quietly and listen to the bell. If you want to, you can think about your new Kindness Pal and imagine yourself doing something kind for him or her.*

Ring the bell or chime. *Thanks for a great class, everyone.*

Week 16
Feelings Game

MINDFULNESS PRACTICE: Flower and Bubble Breaths

OBJECTIVES: Help children name their feelings.

Help children learn to recognize those feelings in others.

Practice kindness.

PREPARE: A bell or chime

Marleigh is Mindful by Linda Ryden

Write different emotions on index cards or just use a list. For this age group, try to keep the words fairly simple, but make sure there are enough words for everyone to have a turn.

Sample Word List: Happy, sad, lonely, scared, angry, tired, nervous, worried, excited, bored, shy, embarrassed, calm, peaceful, relaxed, cheerful, silly, frustrated, proud, annoyed

Your Kindness Pals list and Talking Object

As you and your students have noticed, there are a lot of ways to do mindful breathing! Today we are going to learn two more practices to help students stay calm when they are feeling big emotions like anxiety or frustration. Feel free to make up your own!

Mindfulness Practice

1. **Introduce Flower Breaths and Bubble Breaths**

    Say: *Today we're going to learn two mindful breathing practices that can help you to calm down or focus when you are feeling excited or angry or nervous or frustrated or whatever big emotion you are having.*

    Flower Breaths: *Hold up your finger and pretend that it is a flower. As you breathe in, imagine that you are smelling the flower, as you breathe out, imagine that you are blowing the petals away.*

Bubble Breaths: *Imagine that you have a little bubble wand. Breathe in and then as you breathe out imagine that you are blowing air through the bubble wand to make little bubbles in the air.*

Let's try these for our Mindful Moment. We can do three Flower Breaths and three Bubble Breaths.

2. Mindfulness Practice

Invite today's Mindfulness Helper (MH) to come to the front of the class to sit next to you on a chair.

Prompt the MH to say: *"Let's get into our mindful bodies; Let's close our eyes or look down; Let's take some deep breaths."*

Have the MH lead the class in doing the new breaths.

Say: *In a moment you will hear the sound of the bells and that will mean that it is time to open your eyes or look up. So just get ready for that.*

Ask the MH to ring the bell.

If needed, ask the MH to choose a classmate to turn the lights on.

Ask the MH to return to their seat.

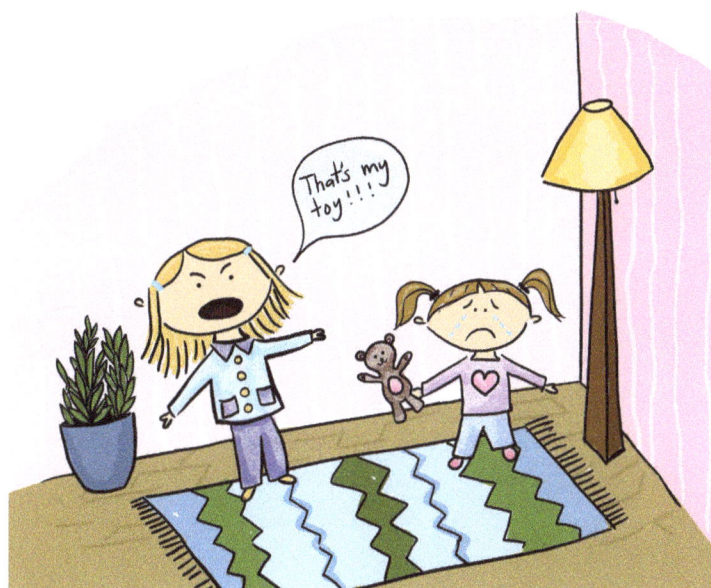

Read and Discuss

Marleigh is Mindful

Say: *Today let's see who has practiced Flower Breathing in* Marleigh is Mindful. *It's Josie and Cybbie!*

Read the two pages on Josie and Cybbie and Flower Breathing.

Ask:

- When do Josie and Cybbie do Flower Breathing? How does it help them?
- How do you think Flower Breathing or Bubble Breathing could help you?

Gratitude Practice

Repeat the "Tell me something good" lesson from last week.

Say: *I'm going to ask you to think of a little good thing in your life and raise your hand. When I call on you we'll all sing "tell me something good," and then you will.*

Call on whomever raises their hand and **say or sing**: "[Child's Name], tell me something good…"

Try to leave enough time for everyone to share. Remind the kids to focus on the little good things.

Activity: The Feelings Game

1. Introduce the Feelings Game.

Say: *Today we are going to be talking about our feelings. We're going to be playing the Feelings Game. Does anybody know how to play a game called charades? Usually you act out the names of books or movies. Today we are going to act out feelings.*

Ask: *Can somebody give me an example of a feeling or an emotion?*

Take a few answers.

2. **Play the Game.**

   Game Guidelines:

   - Most kids will want a turn but some won't.
   - Don't force anyone to have a turn, but make sure that everyone gets the option.
   - Talk about how our voices, bodies, and faces reflect our feelings.

   Say: *I'm going to choose a volunteer and I'm going to whisper a feelings word into their ear. Then he or she is going to say the words:*

   "Today is Tuesday" (or whatever day it is) as if they are feeling that way.

   Demonstrate: Demonstrate by showing one of the feelings yourself.

   Say: *Volunteers can use their faces, the tone of their voice, and their bodies to show the feeling.*

   Then you can raise your hands and try to guess what word they are acting out. Ready to try it?

Kindness Pals

Do the Kindness Pals activity as before.

Closing Words: *Let's have a nice quiet moment with the bell. You can close your eyes or leave them open, but let's sit quietly and listen to the bell. If you want to, you can think about your new Kindness Pal and imagine yourself doing something kind for him or her.*

Ring the bell or chime. *Thanks for a great class, everyone.*

Week 17
Finding Your Feelings

MINDFULNESS PRACTICE: Straw Breathing

OBJECTIVE: Help children locate where they feel emotions in their bodies.

PREPARE:
A bell or chime

Your Kindness Pals list

Copies of the "Finding Your Feelings" Worksheet

Optional: Talking Object

This lesson helps children continue to learn to tune into their bodies and recognize cues to take care of their emotions. We introduce the important ideas that (1) we all feel our emotions in our bodies in unique ways that we can learn to recognize, and (2) if we can increase our awareness of the physical sensations in our bodies and treat them as early warning signs, we increase our ability to recognize and take care of our emotions before they overwhelm us.

Mindfulness Practice

1. **Practice mindful breathing.**

   Invite today's Mindfulness Helper (MH) to come to the front of the class to sit next to you on a chair (or next to you on the floor).

   Say: *Let's all be happy for _____. (sign language applause)*

   Say: *Today we're going to try Straw Breathing again. We're going to pretend that we have a little, tiny straw - like you would have in a juice box. We're going to pretend to put the straw in our mouth, and breathe in through our nose, and then pretend that we are breathing out through the little straw. We're going to see how long we can make that out-breath or exhale last. I'll go first.*

   Demonstrate and have the kids count how long you hold your exhale. Be sure to do it comfortably, we don't want to exaggerate the exhale to a point of discomfort.

Prompt the MH to say: "Let's get into our mindful bodies. Let's close our eyes or look down. Choose the kind of breaths you want to take. Now let's take three deep breaths."

Wait a few moments.

Say: *Now take a deep breath, and listen for the sound of the bell. Try to listen to the whole sound of the bell. Open your eyes when you cannot hear it anymore.*

Ask the MH to ring the bell and return to their seat.

Activity: Feelings and Sensations

1. **Talk about emotions.**

   Say: *Remember last time when we played the Feelings Game? Today we are going to be talking about our feelings. When we are talking about the feelings in our hearts we can also call them emotions. If you start to pay close attention you will notice that you can feel emotions in your body. Let's start by talking about being angry. Can I have a volunteer to come up and show us what anger feels like?*

   Choose someone to demonstrate feeling angry or demonstrate it yourself. Ask them to use their whole body and their voice to say: "I'm so angry!"

   Ask the class to notice what they could see in the volunteer's body. For example, they might notice clenched fists, a scrunched up face, fast breathing or held breath, stomping feet.

   Ask the volunteer to describe where they could feel the anger in their body.

   Ask for another volunteer to demonstrate feeling sad. Again ask the class to comment on what they noticed and ask the volunteer to describe where in their body he or she was feeling the sadness.

2. Feeling emotions in our bodies

Following is a script you can read to your students to help them notice where and how they feel emotions as physical sensations in their bodies.

Say: *Let's get back into our mindful bodies. Let's close our eyes or look down and take a deep breath. I am going to describe some different things and I want you to try to notice what you feel in your body. I am going to ask you some questions, but I don't want you to answer me out loud. You are going to think your answers inside your mind. You can imagine that your answer is in a thought bubble above your head. Ready?*

Imagine that you wake up in the morning and you remember that it is your birthday. How do you feel? Where do you notice that feeling in your body? Point to wherever you feel it in your body. It's okay if you don't feel anything.

Imagine that you smell pancakes cooking. How do you feel? Where do you notice that feeling in your body? Point to wherever you feel it in your body. It's okay if you don't feel anything.

Imagine that you are rushing by and you accidentally knock over the stack of pancakes and they fall all over the floor. How do you feel? Where do you notice that feeling in your body? Point to wherever you feel it in your body. It's okay if you don't feel anything.

Imagine that your brother laughs and calls you clumsy. How do you feel? Where do you notice that feeling in your body? Point to wherever you feel it in your body. It's okay if you don't feel anything.

Imagine that your mom says that you can have a birthday donut instead and she puts a candle in a donut and lets you blow out the candle while she sings "Happy Birthday" to you. How do you feel? Where do you notice that feeling in your body? Point to wherever you feel it in your body. It's okay if you don't feel anything.

Let's take one more deep breath and then let's open our eyes.

3. Share observations.

You can share your own observations, especially if it seems like the children are having trouble articulating what they noticed. This can be a very subtle practice at first.

> **NOTE:** *Remember that anything the children feel is fine. Maybe they don't like pancakes or birthdays. Be sure to be respectful of their feelings.*

Say*: Let's share what we noticed happening in our bodies. When you woke up and realized it was your birthday, how did you feel? What emotion were you feeling? Could you feel it in your body? Where did you feel it?* **Let them share**.

Now, how did you feel when you came downstairs and saw the pancakes? Could you feel it in your body? Where did you feel it? **Let them share**.

How did you feel when you knocked over the pancakes? Could you feel it in your body? Where did you feel it? **Let them share**.

How did you feel when your brother was mean to you? Could you feel it in your body? Where did you feel it? **Let them share**.

And how did you feel when your mother said you could have a donut with a candle in it? Could you feel it in your body? Where did you feel it? **Let them share.**

Activity: Drawing

Hand out copies of the "Finding Your Feelings" worksheet.

Use the "Finding Your Feelings" worksheet to help illustrate the lesson.

Instruct: *Draw a picture of yourself feeling happy or sad or angry, and see if you can point to the parts of your body where you might notice that feeling.*

Keep noticing.

Say: *For the rest of the day, try to notice what is happening in your body when you have different emotions.*

You might suggest:

- Maybe you will be playing a game after school. If you win the game, notice how you feel and see if you can point to that place on your body.
- If you lose the game, notice how you feel.
- If you get one of your favorite things for dinner, notice how you feel.
- If you get something for dinner that you don't really like, notice how you feel.

Kindness Pals

Do the Kindness Pals activity as before.

Closing Words: *Let's have a nice quiet moment with the bell. You can close your eyes or leave them open, but let's sit quietly and listen to the bell. If you want to, you can think about your new Kindness Pal and imagine yourself doing something kind for him or her.*

Ring the bell or chime. *Thanks for a great class, everyone.*

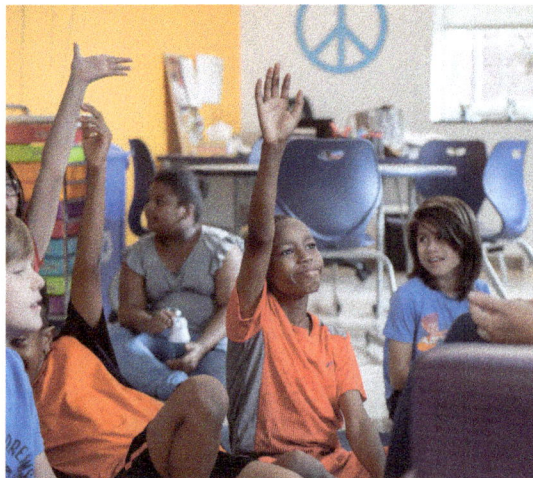

Week 18
Mindful Listening Challenge

MINDFULNESS PRACTICE: Mindful Listening Challenge

OBJECTIVES: Practice mindful listening.

Practice gratitude.

Practice kindness.

PREPARE: A bell or chime

Objects that make sounds, such as: scissors, a bell, a jar of marbles, a wind-up toy, a creaky chair, your footsteps, a jar of pencils, a stack of paper—use your imagination.

Commonalities Worksheet

Your Kindness Pal list

Optional: Talking Object

In this lesson, we give students another way to practice noticing how emotions and sensations relate to each other, involving not only our minds but our whole bodies in the mindful listening practice. When we listen with our whole bodies, we are able to fully hear another person and to understand our own responses more clearly.

Mindfulness practice

Say: *Today when we do our mindfulness practice we are going to be focusing on listening to the sounds around us.*

Invite today's Mindfulness Helper (MH) to come to the front of the class to sit next to you on a chair (or next to you on the floor).

Say: *Let's all be happy for _____.* (sign language applause)

Say: *Today, you will practice listening to sounds in the classroom with your eyes closed or covered up… You can guess what the sounds are in your mind, but please wait until the activity is over to share those guesses.*

Invite the MH to help the class get set up for the lesson.

Say: *Let's all be happy for* _____. *(sign language applause)*

Prompt the MH to say: "Let's get into our mindful bodies. Let's close our eyes or look down. Let's take three deep breaths."

Say: *Now just let your breath settle back into its natural rhythm. Just breathe and listen to my voice while you keep your eyes closed.*

Today we are going to practice our mindful listening again. I am going to make some sounds and every time you hear one of these sounds I want you to raise your hand and then put it down again. Try really hard not to peek, just try to hear the sound. If you want to guess what the sound is go ahead, but try to keep that guess inside your mind until we are done. Let's begin.

Walk around the room making the sounds but leaving plenty of time in between the sounds for quiet. You can do this for as long as the children seem to be able to hold their attention—probably a maximum of 3 or 4 minutes.

Say: *Now take a deep breath, and listen for the sound of the bell. Try to listen to the whole sound of the bell. Open your eyes when you cannot hear it anymore.*

Ask the MH to ring the bell when the mindful breathing is complete.

Ask the MH to return to their seat.

Extension: you can repeat this with other sounds, perhaps using your phone to play a series of sounds and see if the kids can identify them.

Discuss and Reflect

Ask the children what sounds they heard.

Invite them to share their guesses.

How did you feel when you heard [name a sound]. Where did you feel it?

Did you want to peek and see what the sound was? What did that feel like? Where did you feel it?

Activity: Commonalities

This activity will help your students continue to get to know and appreciate each other.

Say: *Today we are going to do a little activity that will help us get to know each other better. We will find out what we have in common and what is different about us.*

Ask students to pair up with their Kindness Pals.

Ask the students to interview each other about the questions on the worksheet.

> *NOTE:* **Do not have children write things down—this is a listening exercise.**

Come back together as a group.

Ask students to raise their hand if both partners had everything in common.

Ask students to raise their hand if the partners like the same animal, the same ice cream, and so on.

Notice all of the similarities in the class

Kindness Pals

Do the Kindness Pals activity as before.

Closing Words: *Let's have a nice quiet moment with the bell. You can close your eyes or leave them open, but let's sit quietly and listen to the bell. If you want to, you can think about your new Kindness Pal and imagine yourself doing something kind for him or her.*

Ring the bell or chime. *Thanks for a great class, everyone.*

Week 19
Visualization

MINDFULNESS PRACTICE: Visualization

OBJECTIVES: Practice mindful breathing.

Learn the skill of visualization to calm down and focus.

Practice kindness.

PREPARE: A bell or chime

Marleigh is Mindful by Linda Ryden

Your Kindness Pals list

Copies of the Visualization Worksheet

Optional: Talking Object

In this lesson, we introduce Visualization, another way to notice our emotions and physical sensations in a new and peaceful scenario. Visualization is also a fun way to practice mindfulness that the children really enjoy! Focusing our minds on a peaceful place can help us to calm down, to think about our senses, and to really settle ourselves into the moment, even if it is in our imagination.

You can tailor this lesson to the specific needs of your class. If you have students with disabilities that might make using some of the "five senses" challenging, you can change the visualization guidance to meet their specific needs.

Mindfulness Practice

Note: There are lots of ways to do today's Visualization practice. We've provided a script here to get you started. You can ask the kids to imagine a peaceful place, as we've done here, or a land made of candy, outerspace, a beach, and so on. Try to keep the structure of using your five senses.

Invite today's Mindfulness Helper (MH) to come to the front of the class to sit next to you on a chair (or next to you on the floor).

Say: *Let's all be happy for _____.* *(sign language applause)*

Prompt the MH to say: "Let's get into our mindful bodies. Let's close our eyes or look down. Let's take three deep breaths."

Guide the children through a visualization exercise.

Say: *Today we are going to be thinking about a park. Try to picture in your mind a park, either one that you have visited in real life, or one that you create in your imagination.*

Give the students a moment to think.

Say: *Now take a look around at your park. What does the sky look like? Is it blue and clear, or dark and cloudy? What does the grass look like? Are there trees? How many? How big are they? Are there any squirrels? Is there a playground? Is there a slide? Swings? Is there a basketball hoop? What else? Take another look around to see what you might have missed.*

What sounds do you hear at your park? Do you hear birds? Children playing? Do you hear people talking or the sounds of traffic? What else do you hear?

What does it smell like at your park? Can you smell flowers? Are you having a snack that smells good?

What can you feel at the park? Can you touch the bark of a tree? Can you feel the leaf of a flower?

What does it feel like in your heart to be at your park? Notice that for a moment.

Now we are going to travel back to this peaceful place, right here in our classroom.

In a moment you will hear the sound of the bells. That will mean that it is time to open your eyes, so just get ready for that.

Ask the MH to ring the bell when the exercise is complete.

Ask the MH to return to their seat.

Discuss

Ask some children to share a few details about their parks.

You might want to ask first about sights, then sounds, then smells, and so on, so that each child gets to share a detail.

Read and Discuss

Marleigh is Mindful

Say: *Today let's see who does a Visualization Practice in* Marleigh is Mindful. *It's Malachi!! Let's hear about Malachi's experience.*

Read the two pages on Malachi and Visualization.

Ask*:*

- When Malachi has trouble falling asleep, what does he do?
- When could you use a Visualization practice like the one we did today?

Kindness Pals

Do the Kindness Pal activity as before.

If there is not enough time for sharing, you can skip that, but be sure to give the students new Kindness Pals.

Closing Words: *Let's have a nice quiet moment with the bell. You can close your eyes or leave them open, but let's sit quietly and listen to the bell. If you want to, you can think about your new Kindness Pal and imagine yourself doing something kind for him or her.*

Ring the bell or chime. *Thanks for a great class, everyone*

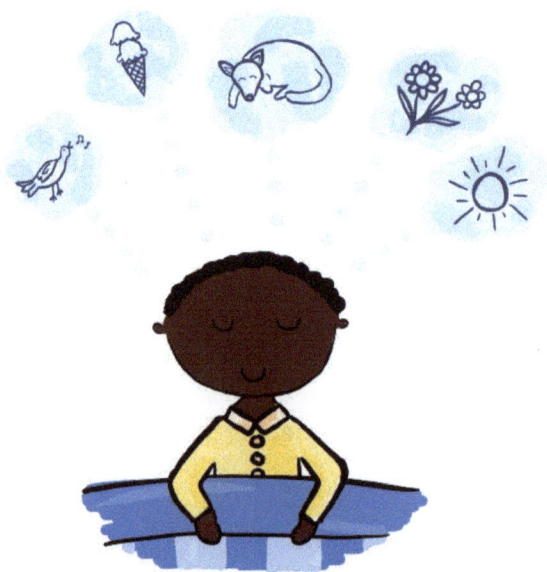

UNIT 4:
Brain Science

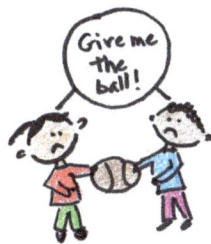

stimulus

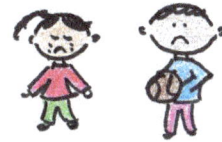

Reaction

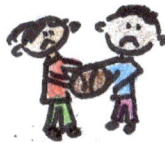

Stimulus

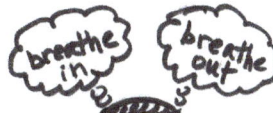

Mindfulness

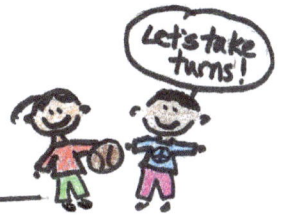

Response

Week 20
Rosie's Brain

MINDFULNESS PRACTICE: Take Five, Wave Breathing and Gravity Hands

OBJECTIVES: Learn about three parts of your brain.

Practice kindness.

PREPARE: A bell or chime

Rosie's Brain by Linda Ryden

Your Kindness Pals list

Optional: Brainy the Puppet

Optional: Talking Object

Our brains are complex and quite amazing parts of our bodies. In this curriculum, we offer a very simplified look at how our brains work in order to help children understand why we practice mindfulness and how it helps. We focus on two important components of the limbic system, the amygdala and the hippocampus, and also on the integrating portions of the brain's cortex, the prefrontal cortex.

To make these concepts accessible to young learners, we'll be reading a book called *Rosie's Brain*. In this book, students will be introduced to three characters representing the amygdala, hippocampus and prefrontal cortex.

We will start with mindfulness practice in which students can choose the practice that works best for them.

Mindfulness Practice

Invite today's Mindfulness Helper (MH) to come to the front of the class to sit next to you on a chair (or next to you on the floor).

Say: *Let's all be happy for _____. (sign language applause)*

Say: *Today when the Mindfulness Helper asks us to take deep breaths, you can do Take Five Breathing, Wave breathing, Gravity Hands, or you can create a new way to take deep breaths. Remember that whatever you do needs to be calm and quiet to go along with your calm, quiet, deep breaths.*

Prompt the MH to say: "Let's get into our mindful bodies. Let's close our eyes or look down. Let's take three deep breaths." Students can choose their own practice.

Say: *After you are done taking your deep breaths, let your breath settle back into its natural rhythm. Just breathe in and out normally. Put a hand on your tummy and see if you can make the rest of your body so still that the only thing that you feel moving is your breath.*

Wait about 30 seconds.

Say: *In a moment you will hear the sound of the bell. When you hear that sound, it will be time to open your eyes if they are closed.*

Ask the MH to ring the bell and return to their seat

Read and Discuss

Prepare to read *Rosie's Brain*.

Say: *Today we are going to start learning about our brains. Our brains are amazing and complicated and learning a little bit about how they work can be really helpful. We're going to start out by reading a story about a little girl named Rosie who gets really mad when she doesn't get what she wants.*

Read the story. Stopping along the way, ask these questions:

- Why was Rosie angry?
- What did her Amygdala (Amy) want her to do?
- Was Amy's idea (smashing the piano) a good one?
- How did her Hippocampus (Miss Pickles) help her?
- How did her PFC help her?
- Can you think of another way to solve Rosie's problem?

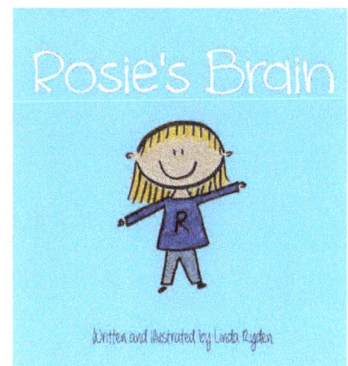

Activity: Walk Stop Wiggle Sit (WSWS)

Introduce the game: *In Rosie's Brain, Rosie used mindful breathing to calm her amygdala down and put her PFC in charge. When our PFC is in charge it's much easier to think and make good decisions.*

Today we're going to play a brain game that challenges our PFC to focus on one thing.

Here's how to play. There are many levels of this game.

Give directions to play Walk, Stop, Wiggle, Sit:

- We're going to play the game without talking so that everyone can hear the directions.
- You won't get "out" if you make a mistake. Just keep trying.
- Make sure that you are not talking and that you are not touching anybody else.

For this first round,
- When I say Walk, you are going to walk.
- When I say Stop, you are going to stop.
- When I say Wiggle, you are going to wiggle.
- When I say Sit, you are going to sit down. Got it?

Level 1:

Walk = Walk

Stop = Stop

Wiggle = Wiggle

Sit = Sit

Try it a few times, changing the order and timing of the commands.

Level 2:

Say: *This time we're going to switch things up. When I say Walk you are going to Stop. When I say Stop you are going to Walk. When I say Wiggle you are still going to Wiggle. When I say Sit you are still going to Sit. Okay?*

Walk = Stop

Stop = Walk

Wiggle = Wiggle

Sit = Sit

Try it a few times, changing the order and timing of the commands.

Level 3:

Say: Okay now I'm going to make it a little harder. This time when I say Walk you are going to Stop. When I say Stop you are going to Walk. When I say Wiggle you are going to Sit and when I saw Sit you are going to Wiggle.

Walk = Stop

Stop = Walk

Wiggle = Sit

Sit = Wiggle

Try it a few times, changing the order and timing of the commands.

> *NOTE: You can make many more variations of this game - adding more levels, letting students lead the game, adding in different movements, etc. Have fun! Start out with a few levels and then add on more each time you play it. You'll be playing again in a couple of weeks.*

Kindness Pals

Do the Kindness Pal activity as before.

If there is not enough time for sharing, you can skip that, but be sure to give the students new Kindness Pals.

Closing Words: *Let's have a nice quiet moment with the bell. You can close your eyes or leave them open, but let's sit quietly and listen to the bell. If you want to, you can think about your new Kindness Pal and imagine yourself doing something kind for him or her.*

Ring the bell or chime. *Thanks for a great class, everyone.*

Week 21
Learn About Your Amygdala with Brainy

MINDFULNESS PRACTICE: Take Five

OBJECTIVES: Learn about how the amygdala operates.

                          Practice kindness.

PREPARE: A bell or chime

                          Copies of the Amygdala Worksheet (in the
                          Resource Section)

                          Video of Dr. Daniel Siegel's Model of the
                          Brain. Watch this before class: **for the teacher,
                          not the students** http://www.drdansiegel.
                          com/resources/everyday_mindsight_tools/

                          Review diagram of the brain (see Resource
                          Section)

                          Your Kindness Pals list

                          Optional: Brainy the Puppet

                          Optional: Talking Object

This lesson is written to include Peace of Mind's puppet called Brainy. We
have designed Brainy to complement the lessons and stories presented here.
The children we work with love Brainy, and it really seems to help them learn.
However, you can do this lesson without Brainy by using your hand to make the
model of the brain as in the video featuring Dr. Siegel. Wherever it says "Brainy
the Puppet" below, please feel free to substitute your hand if you prefer.

NOTE FROM LINDA: *This is really a personal choice depending on
your comfort level and your personality. If you enjoy doing funny voices you
can have Brainy talk - you can have "Amy" have a separate voice. Feel free to
make this your own. I usually don't have Brainy talk like a traditional puppet
but you can make it the way it feels right to you.*

Mindfulness Practice

Invite today's Mindfulness Helper (MH) to come to the front of the class to sit next to you on a chair (or next to you on the floor).

Say: *Let's all be happy for _____. (sign language applause)*

Prompt the MH to say: "Let's get into our mindful bodies. Let's close our eyes or look down. Let's take **five** deep breaths." Remind the children how to do Take Five breathing.

Now take a deep breath, and listen for the sound of the bell. Try to listen to the whole sound of the bell. Open your eyes or look up when you cannot hear it anymore.

Ask the MH to ring the bell and return to their seat.

Brain Science

Introduce Brainy.

Use Dr. Daniel Siegel's hand model of the brain and Brainy the puppet (or your hand) to explain how the amygdala and the prefrontal cortex come into play when we are angry. (See above.)

Remember, DO NOT show Dan Siegel's video to the class.

You might say:

Today I'd like to introduce you to my friend Brainy. Brainy is going to help us learn about our brains. Do you remember the three parts of your brain that we learned about last time when we read the book Rosie's Brain?

That's right, we learned about the Amygdala, the Hippocampus, and the Prefrontal Cortex! Today with Brainy's help we are going to learn more about our Amygdala.

Hold up Brainy in the closed position (fingers folded down over your thumb) in the shape of the hand model.

Can you do this with your hand? Tuck your thumb inside and then fold your fingers over your thumb. Now your hand looks a little bit like your brain.

Hold Brainy up next to your head.

The first part of the brain we're going to learn about is called the Amygdala. (Ah-mig-duh-la) The amygdala is the little part of your brain inside here. (point to your thumb) *What is the Amygdala called in* <u>Rosie's Brain</u>*? That's right - Amy!*

Lift your fingers to show the tucked-in thumb.

The amygdala has a really important job. It's job is to keep you safe. It is always watching out for danger and getting ready to protect you. It's like your brain's little security guard. Sometimes the amygdala is really good at its job and sometimes it needs a little help.

Has this ever happened to you? You were about to cross the street when you heard a car coming. What do you do? (take some answers)

Do you think it would be a good idea to stand there and think for a while about what you should do? No! You need to act fast. That is something that the amygdala is great at. The amygdala doesn't stop and think - the amygdala just reacts. (open your Brainy so that the amygdala is out and your fingers are stretched back) *So when your amygdala hears that car coming it immediately tells you to jump back up on the sidewalk. Phew! Great job, Amygdala!*

Here's another example: What do you do if somebody yells "Duck!"? (take some answers)

That's right - you would cover your head and maybe get down low. Why do you think you do that? That's right - Amygdala! If the amygdala thinks something is flying at your head it isn't going to stop and think about what to do. It is going to protect you. Thanks Amygdala!

But sometimes the amygdala gets a little confused. Sometimes the amygdala thinks you are in danger when you are really just disappointed or frustrated or mad.

In the story <u>Rosie's Brain</u>, why was Rosie angry? That's right - she didn't want to go to her piano lesson because she wanted to play frisbee with her friend Henry.

Was Rosie in danger? No! But Amy thought she was because Rosie was angry.

So how did Amy react? That's right - she yelled at her mom, threw her bagel on the floor, stomped upstairs and slammed the door.

Ask: Has this ever happened to you?

Maybe you were hoping to have ice cream after dinner but then your grown up tells you that you can't have any. How would you feel? Do you think you might yell, "No!! That's not fair! I WANT ICE CREAM!"

How about this? You are playing with Legos with your friend and they take some of the pieces you are using. How would you feel? Do you think you might say, "Hey give those back!! THOSE ARE MINE!!!" Do you think you might want to grab the Legos back?

Can you think of a time when your amygdala thought you were in danger but maybe you were just mad, or frustrated or disappointed because you didn't get what you wanted?

Take some answers.

We each might have different reactions but those are examples of your amygdala thinking you are in danger when you aren't. When your amygdala thinks you're in danger it doesn't stop to think about what to do. It just reacts. And sometimes that reaction doesn't really help. Sometimes it makes things a lot worse. Do you think you're going to get ice cream after yelling about it? Probably not. Do you think if you grab Legos from your friend that they are going to want to play with you? Maybe not.

So the more that we understand how the amygdala works the easier it is for us to help.

Fight, Flight or Freeze

The amygdala only has three ways of reacting when it thinks you are in danger. They all start with the letter "F".

Fight

When you get mad at your little sister for ripping up your new drawing and you feel like hitting her, that is one of the amygdala's reactions. Can anybody guess what that word that starts with "F" is? (Take some guesses)

It's "Fight". When the amygdala thinks you are in danger it might think that it would be helpful to fight. If you were really in danger that might be a good idea but most of the time it isn't.

Flight

When I see a mouse my amygdala usually wants me to run away. That is another reaction that the amygdala has - we call it "Flight". It doesn't mean that you can fly when you get mad! But it's a word that means to run away. Sometimes that can be helpful but sometimes it's not a good idea.

The third reaction you might have seen when you have surprised a squirrel. Usually if a squirrel sees you it is scared because you are a big human. So a squirrel isn't going to put up his little dukes and fight you. What do you think the squirrel will do? Run? That's right - flight!

Freeze

The other thing a squirrel might do is freeze. It might freeze in one place in the hopes that you won't see it. That's the squirrel's amygdala at work!

Rosie's Brain

What choice did Amy make in <u>Rosie's Brain</u>? That's right - Fight! She wanted Rosie to yell and throw stuff and even smash the piano into a million pieces!

So the amygdala's three choices are Fight, Flight, and Freeze. That's it. That's all the amygdala can do. Sometimes those are really helpful, good ideas and sometimes they make things worse.

Your amygdala feels scared sometimes too. Your amygdala might tell you not to jump off the diving board or not to raise your hand in class to answer a hard question.

*Your amygdala wants to take care of you, to protect you. But, if we **only** listened to our amygdala, we wouldn't be very happy. We'd be in fights with people all of the time and we wouldn't do anything that we are scared to do, even really fun things like learning how to ride a bike or learning how to swim.*

So sometimes we have to take care of the amygdala. And luckily we have already learned how to do that? Can anybody think of something we have learned so far in Peace class that would help us to take care of the amygdala?

Take some answers.

That's right - mindful breathing! Taking slow deep breaths - like Take Five Breathing or Wave Breaths or Tummy Breaths (or whatever else you have been practicing) can be a great way to send a message to the amygdala that we are not in danger and don't need their help right now.

So the next time you feel yourself getting angry you can say, "That's okay, Amygdala! I'm not in danger" and you can take some deep breaths. See what happens!

Discuss

Ask: *Can you think of a time when your amygdala tried to help you and it helped?* (take some answers)

Can you think of a time when your amygdala tried to help you and it made things worse? (take some answers)

Activity: Drawing

Pass out the Amygdala worksheet.

Invite the students to think of a time when their amygdala tried to help them.

Say: *Let's draw about it!*

Next time we'll learn more about some other parts of our brains.

Kindness Pals

Do the Kindness Pal activity as before.

If there is not enough time for sharing, you can skip that, but be sure to give the students new Kindness Pals.

Closing Words: *Let's have a nice quiet moment with the bell. You can close your eyes or leave them open, but let's sit quietly and listen to the bell. If you want to, you can think about your new Kindness Pal and imagine yourself doing something kind for him or her.*

Ring the bell or chime. *Thanks for a great class, everyone.*

Week 22
Learn about Your PFC With Brainy

MINDFULNESS PRACTICE: Take Five, Gravity Hands, Wave Breathing, Straw Breathing.

OBJECTIVE: Learn about the role of the prefrontal cortex.

PREPARE:

A bell or chime

Your Kindness Pals list

Optional: Brainy the Puppet

Optional: Talking Object

In the last lesson, we learned about the role of the amygdala. This week's focus is on the prefrontal cortex (PFC), the part of the brain that helps us to make good decisions about how to respond in challenging situations. Students learn how mindfulness can help to put the PFC back in charge when the amygdala has taken over. We'll start this lesson with student-choice mindfulness practice.

Mindfulness Practice

Invite today's Mindfulness Helper (MH) to come to the front of the class to sit next to you on a chair (or next to you on the floor).

Say: *Let's all be happy for _____.* (sign language applause)

Say: *Today the Mindfulness Helper can choose what we will do. We can do Take Five, Gravity Hands, Wave Breathing, Straw Breathing. What will it be?*

Wait for the Mindfulness Helper to choose.

Prompt the MH to say: "Let's get into our mindful bodies. Let's close our eyes or look down. Let's take three deep _____ breaths."

Say: *Now listen for the sound of the bell. Try to listen to the whole sound of the bell. Open your eyes or look up when you cannot hear it anymore.*

Ask the MH to ring the bell when the mindful breathing is complete and return to their seat.

114 | All Rights Reserved. Please do not copy or share without express written permission from Peace of Mind Inc. | https://TeachPeaceofMind.org

1. Review last week's lesson.

Say: *Let's say "hello" again to our friend Brainy! Does anyone remember what we learned about Brainy last time? Does anybody remember the funny name of this part? (Point to your thumb/the amygdala.) That's right, it's the amygdala!*

Does anybody remember what the amygdala does?

Take a few answers.

That's right, the amygdala tries to keep us safe. The amygdala is like the security guard of the brain. Does anybody remember my nickname for the amygdala?

Take a few answers.

That's right - Amy! Today we're going to meet another part of our brain.

Fold your fingers back down.

*This part (**pointing to your folded-over fingers or Brainy's front**) is called the Prefrontal Cortex. You can call it the PFC for short. Your Prefrontal Cortex is the part of your brain that helps you to make decisions. It thinks things over and imagines what will happen. It's like the boss of your brain.*

Choose a volunteer to demonstrate with you.

Ask the student to do a series of actions like: stand up, stand on one leg, stand on the other leg, turn around in a circle, find something in the room and bring it to you, and so on.

Make the tasks a little more complicated each time - like find something red and walk over to it without stepping on any lines on the floor or something like that.

Say: *(Student's name) just used their prefrontal cortex! They made decisions, sent messages to other parts of the brain, figured out problems, etc.*

One of the reasons that they were able to do all of those things is because they feel pretty calm right now. Their PFC is able to really think well.

2. Don't forget about Amy!

Say: *Do you remember in Rosie's Brain how Amy was trying to help Rosie but was really making things worse? What part of Rosie's Brain actually had good ideas to solve the problem? That's right - the PFC! But the PFC couldn't think of those great ideas while Amy was screaming and yelling. When Rosie took some deep breaths, Amy was able to quiet down and take a nap and the PFC could be in charge again and think.*

Usually our PFC is in charge of our brains. Your PFC is probably in charge right now if you are feeling pretty calm and you are able to listen to me.

But when we feel angry like Rosie did, it can feel like we've flipped our lid (flip your fingers up exposing the amygdala). It can feel like our amygdala is in charge, and we can't think very well because our Prefrontal Cortex or PFC is no longer working. It's like the amygdala shuts down the PFC and takes over the brain. And remember, the amygdala only has three choices - Fight, Flight, or Freeze.

3. How does knowing all this help us?

You might ask: How does knowing about our brains help us?

Say: *When we take our deep breaths and take care of our anger, it helps to bring our Prefrontal Cortex back in charge (fold your fingers down slowly). It can take a little while to work, but once we have our lids back on we can think about what we want to do. We have choices.*

If you were making a block tower or playing your favorite game and a parent called you for dinner, do you have any choices in how you respond besides flipping your lid?

You might ask for a couple more minutes, ask if you could just finish this round of the game, or maybe just realize that dinner is ready and that your game or tower will still be there when you get back.

Do you see how your PFC helps you see that you have choices and sometimes what your amygdala wants you to do isn't always the best idea?

The next time you get angry, see if you can remember that this is your amygdala talking to you. See if you can use your breathing to help take care of your amygdala.

We like to say that when we get really angry we have flipped our lids. That means that our anger has taken over our brains and that our amygdala is in charge. Did anybody flip your lid this week? (If you can think of an example, it can be powerful to share your own experience.)

When we flip our lids, we feel out of control, and it can be kind of scary. Sometimes we say things or do things that we don't really mean to do. Sometimes we hurt people that we really like or break things. It is not a good feeling. Luckily we have already learned the best way to help us when we flip our lids. Can you guess what that is?

Take a few answers

That's right, it's our mindful breathing! Doing those slow deep breaths we've been practicing, like Take Five, Wave, or your own way of deep breathing, can calm down your amygdala and put your PFC back in charge. When our PFC is in charge, we can make some good decisions.

Activity: WSWS Game

Play the Walk, Stop, Wiggle, Sit game again. Start at the first level and add more variations and complications.

You can try to make it harder by giving one command "Walk" but doing something else with your body like sit or wiggle.

Remember to point out that this game is challenging to the PFC because it is calling on a lot of different parts of the brain, the memory and trying to stay focused.

Invite students to imagine how hard this would be if you were really angry or upset!

Kindness Pals

Do the Kindness Pal activity as before.

If there is not enough time for sharing, you can skip that, but be sure to give the students new Kindness Pals.

Closing Words: *Let's have a nice quiet moment with the bell. You can close your eyes or leave them open, but let's sit quietly and listen to the bell.   If you want to, you can think about your new Kindness Pal and imagine yourself doing something kind for him or her.*

Ring the bell or chime. *Thanks for a great class, everyone.*

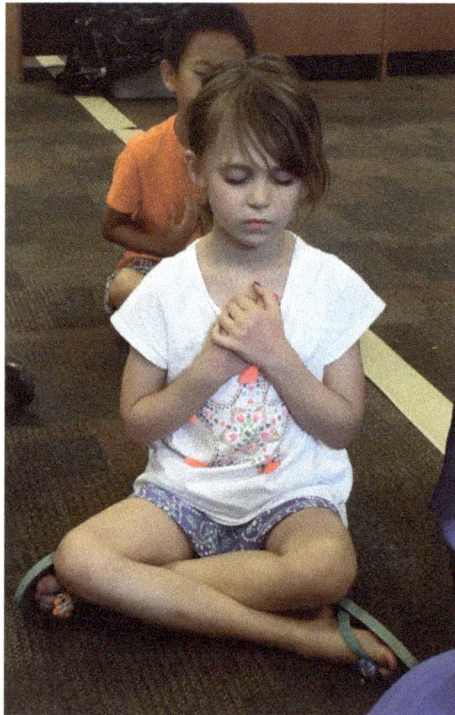

Week 23

Learn about your Hippocampus with Miss Pickles

MINDFULNESS PRACTICE: Blooming Breaths

OBJECTIVES:
Learn about the Hippocampus.

Practice gratitude.

Practice kindness.

PREPARE:
A bell or chime

Marleigh is Mindful by Linda Ryden

Your Kindness Pals list

Optional: Brainy the Puppet

Optional: Talking Object

We start this week with the Tell Me Something Good gratitude practice we first learned in Week 10. This is a practice you can use anytime to help your students focus on what is good in their lives. We'll then learn a new Mindfulness Breathing Practice called Blooming Breaths and learn about the Hippocampus. Have fun!

Gratitude Practice: Tell Me something Good

Say: *I'm going to ask you to think of a little good thing in your life and raise your hand. When I call on you, we'll all sing "tell me something good," and then you will.*

Call on whomever raises their hand and **say or sing**: "[Child's Name], tell me something good…"

Try to leave enough time for everyone to share. Remind the kids to focus on the little good things.

Mindfulness Practice

1. Introduce Blooming Breaths

Blooming Breaths is a mindful breathing practice that was created by one of my students. She had a little pond in her backyard that had water lilies floating in it. She loved the water lilies and the way that they opened up in the mornings and closed up in the evenings. It's fun to give kids lots of different ways to do mindful breathing and adding a gesture helps to remind them of the practice and make it a little more tangible and easier to focus.

Say: *Today we're going to learn a breathing practice called Blooming Breaths. Have you ever seen water lilies? They are those pretty white flowers that float on ponds. Water lilies are interesting because they open every morning and close up again every night. The flowers last for a few days.*

Let's pretend that our hands are like those water lilies. Hold your hands out in front of you with your palms up and then bring your fingers and thumb together. Then open your hands up and spread your fingers and thumb out wide. Slowly open and close your hands imagining that they are like the water lilies. Now let's add some breathing to it. Start with your "water lilies" closed. Then slowly and gently breathe in and open your lilies wide (stretch your fingers). Then slowly and gently breathe out and close your lilies up (fingers and thumbs together). Let's try that a few times slowly together.

Breathing, moving our hands, and thinking about water lilies can be a great way to help us to settle down when we are angry or nervous or having another kind of big emotion. Let's try it now for our "official" Mindful Moment.

2. Mindful Moment

Invite today's Mindfulness Helper (MH) to come to the front of the class to sit next to you on a chair (or next to you on the floor).

Say: *Let's all be happy for _____. (sign language applause)*

Prompt the MH to say: "Let's get into our mindful bodies. Let's close our eyes or look down. Let's take three deep Blooming Breaths."

Ask the MH to ring the bell when the mindful breathing is complete.

Ask the MH to return to their seat.

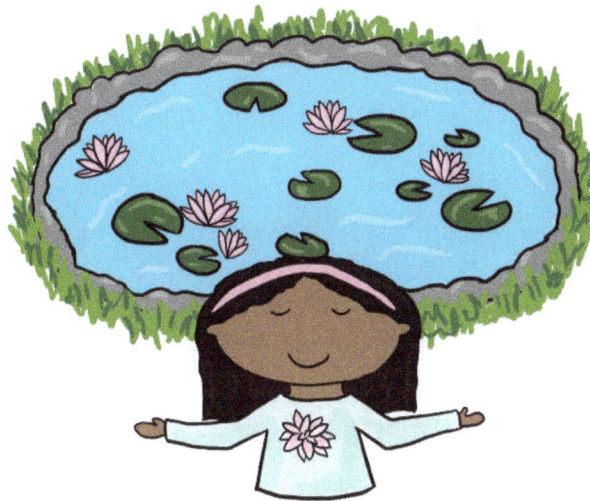

Read and Discuss

Marleigh is Mindful

Say: *Today let's see who does Blooming Breath's in* Marleigh is Mindful. *It's Alexis!! Let's hear about Alexis' experience.*

Read the two pages on Alexis and Blooming Breaths.

Ask*:*

- When Alexis is annoyed at her brother, what does she do to feel better?
- When could you use Blooming Breaths?

Brain Science: Meet the Hippocampus

Say*: In this lesson, we will be adding to our knowledge of the brain by learning about the Hippocampus. Who can remind us of the two parts of the brain we've learned about so far? Can anybody remember what they were called or what they did?* (the amygdala and the prefrontal cortex)

Take some answers.

Review the jobs of the amygdala and the PFC.

You might continue by saying:

Well there are lots of other parts of your brain. Today we are going to learn about the Hippocampus. The hippocampus is like a big storage cabinet or a library inside of your brain. It is the part of the brain that stores all of your memories.

Ask: *Does anybody remember what the Hippocampus is called in <u>Rosie's Brain</u>? That's right - Miss Pickles!*

Ask: *Can anybody tell me what you had for breakfast today?*

Take some answers.

Well that memory was stored in your hippocampus!

Ask some more questions:

- Have you ever been to the beach?
- Eaten a pepper?
- Touched a snake?

Let kids raise their hands if they have done any of those things.

Say: *When I asked those questions, your brains went looking in the hippocampus for the answer. Some of us found it, but some of us didn't because it was not there. Sometimes you forget something and that means that it was a little harder for your hippocampus to find it.*

Activity: Memory Game

In this game, Kindness Pals will ask each other five questions and try to remember the answers. To make this game easier, you can write the questions on the board. To make it more challenging you can ask them to try to remember the questions. You can ask your students if they have any strategies for remembering the questions. Then remind them that they are going to try to remember their Kindness Pal's answers to the questions.

This is a great opportunity to practice mindful listening and make sure that the kids are really listening to each other rather than just focusing on their own answers.

Introduce the game: *Today we're going to play a memory game with our Kindness Pals. I'm going to give you five questions to ask your Kindness Pal and you are going to try to remember their answers.*

Assign this week's Kindness Pals in the usual way.

Say: *Okay so now you are going to sit with your Kindness Pal and ask each other these questions:*

1. *What is your favorite ice cream flavor?*
2. *What is your favorite animal?*
3. *What is your favorite season?*
4. *Do you have a pet?*
5. *What did you have for breakfast?*

Give them 5 or so minutes to play and then bring the group back together to share their answers.

Kindness Pals

If you still have time they can share what they did for their Kindness Pal last week.

Closing Words: *Let's have a nice quiet moment with the bell. You can close your eyes or leave them open, but let's sit quietly and listen to the bell. If you want to, you can think about your new Kindness Pal and imagine yourself doing something kind for him or her.*

Ring the bell or chime. *Thanks for a great class, everyone.*

Week 24
Jonah Flips His Lid

MINDFULNESS PRACTICE: Take Five and Wave Breathing

OBJECTIVES: Learn about using Mindful Breathing to help when you Flip Your Lid.

Practice kindness.

PREPARE: A bell or chime

Your Kindness Pals list

Optional: Brainy the Puppet

Optional: Talking Object

In this lesson, students will have the chance to experience how everything they have been learning applies in practice. Through a story about what happens when kids get angry and "flip their lids," students learn how mindfulness practice can calm them down enough to work things out. This lesson is a bridge to the next Unit on Conflict Resolution. Practicing through skits helps children internalize the lessons and practices so they are available when they are really needed.

Mindfulness Practice

Before you begin, ask the class what kind of breathing they would like to practice today. Let them choose between Take Five, Wave, or Gravity Hands. Everybody can choose which one they want to do. This can be a fun way to keep them excited about the mindfulness practice.

Invite today's Mindfulness Helper (MH) to come to the front of the class to sit next to you on a chair (or next to you on the floor).

Say: *Let's all be happy for _____. (sign language applause)*

Prompt the MH to say: "Let's get into our mindful bodies. Let's close our eyes or look down. Let's (insert whatever they decided to do here.)"

Say: *Now let your breath settle back into its natural rhythm. Just breathe. Put your hand on your belly and try to make your body so still and quiet that the only thing that you can feel moving is your breath.*

Wait a few moments to see how long they can hold this focus.

Say: *Now take a deep breath, and listen for the sound of the bell. Try to listen to the whole sound of the bell. Open your eyes when you cannot hear it anymore.*

Ask the MH to ring the bell and return to their seat

Read and Act Out

1. Introduce the story

Say: *Today we are going to act out a story about a boy who flips his lid. Who can remind us about what it means to "flip your lid"? That's right - it means that when we get mad or frustrated or nervous our amygdala will take over our brain. The amygdala will turn off our PFC and our Hippocampus so that it is hard for us to think and to remember things.*

2. Recruit volunteers to act it out

Recruit Volunteers. You will need five volunteers to act out this story. The characters are Jonah, Amani, Sammy, Jonah's mom or dad, and Happy the dog.

> **NOTE:** *I like to include characters who don't speak for kids who might feel a little less comfortable participating in a speaking role. Feel free to change the names, genders, etc. of these characters to fit the needs of your class.*

Say to the volunteers: *I'm going to read the story out loud and you all are going to act it out. I'll read the lines for your character and if you want to repeat them you can but you don't have to. Try to pretend that you are doing what your character is doing. So if your character is running what will you do?*

Say to the rest of the class: *Before we begin the story, you all have a job to do, too. I want you to watch the story closely and every time you notice that one of the characters is flipping their lid I want you to show me by using the hand model.*

Demonstrate the "flipping your lid" gesture with Brainy or your hand.

Start with Jonah in the middle, Jonah's Mom or Dad and Happy on the left and Amani and Sammy on the right.

3. Read the story

<u>Jonah Flips His Lid</u> by Linda Ryden

Jonah was a very happy boy. He liked to run around with his friends, he liked to walk his dog, he liked to play basketball, he liked to play the piano, and he loved to make pancakes.

Remind the student playing Jonah to mime all of these activities, and do the same for other actors.

His best friend was a girl named Amani.

Amani was a really funny girl. She liked to play guitar, she liked to ice skate, she liked to play baseball, and she liked to read.

Jonah and Amani loved to play together. They played tennis together, they played catch together, they told each other secrets, and they made each other laugh.

Whenever Jonah had a cookie he always shared it with Amani. Whenever Amani had some candy she always shared it with Jonah. They got along perfectly. Well… most of the time…

One day Amani was playing with her other friend Sammy (*Amani should walk over to Sammy*). Sammy was teaching Amani how to bake chocolate chip cookies. He was showing Amani how to crack the eggs so that the shells didn't get into the batter. It was hard and Amani was starting to get frustrated.

Jonah came over to Amani's house to play and was surprised to see Sammy there. He said to Amani, "Come on, Amani, let's go play in the park." Amani said, "Not now. I'm busy."

Jonah was hurt. He felt left out and wanted Amani to play with him. He asked her again, "Come on, Amani. Pleeeeease…" Amani was really bothered now so she shouted, "No! I'm learning how to make cookies! Go away!" And she pointed at the door.

Jonah was really mad now. He didn't like feeling left out and he really didn't like the way she was talking to him. He started to feel his body getting angry. His face felt hot, he was breathing faster and harder, and his hands were balling up into little fists. He wanted to punch something and scream.

He yelled at Amani, "Fine! If you don't want to play with me then we're not friends anymore!" and he slammed the door and he stomped away back to his house.

When Jonah got home his Mom (or Dad) heard him stomping into the house and asked him, "What's wrong, Jonah?" "Everything!" he yelled. "I hate Amani, and I hate Sammy, and I hate cookies!"

His mom said, "Okay, it sounds like you have flipped your lid. Your amygdala is really mad and it has taken over your brain. Do you think it would help to Take Five?"

Jonah didn't really want to but he decided to give it a try. He sat down on the floor with his Mom and he traced his hand and took five deep breaths. After he was done he felt a bit better. He felt like his lid was back on. His Mom gave him some water and he patted his dog Happy.

Meanwhile back at Amani's house, Amani was still trying to crack the eggs but she couldn't concentrate. She felt bad about the mean things she said to Jonah. She was just frustrated and busy. It wasn't Jonah's fault.

Sammy said, "Hey Amani, are you okay?" Amani said, "No. I feel bad about what happened with Jonah." Sammy said, "Why don't you take some deep breaths like we learned at school? I like to do Wave breaths when I get angry or sad." "That's a great idea!" said Amani. The two friends took some deep breaths together. "Now that I'm calm I think I have to go say 'I'm sorry' to Jonah," said Amani. Sammy said, "Yeah, that's a good idea. I'll go with you." So they walked over to Jonah's house together.

Amani knocked on Jonah's door. Jonah opened the door and Amani said, "Jonah, I'm sorry I said those mean things. I guess I flipped my lid."

Jonah said, "I'm sorry too! I didn't mean any of the things I said."

Amani said, "That's okay! Do you want to go play in the park with me and Sammy now?"

Jonah said, "I sure do!"

Jonah put a leash on Happy and they all went to play in the park together.

The End

You might use these questions to spark discussion:

- Why did Jonah flip his lid?
- Did he have a reason to be angry?
- How did he feel when his lid was flipped?
- Could he feel that anger in his body?
- Did his actions make him feel better or worse?
- What did he do to help him calm down?
- Why did Amani flip her lid?
- What part of her brain made her yell at Jonah?
- What did she do to help her calm down?

Kindness Pals

Do the Kindness Pal activity as before.

If there is not enough time for sharing, you can skip that, but be sure to give the students new Kindness Pals.

Closing Words: *Let's have a nice quiet moment with the bell. You can close your eyes or leave them open, but let's sit quietly and listen to the bell. If you want to, you can think about your new Kindness Pal and imagine yourself doing something kind for him or her.*

Ring the bell or chime. *Thanks for a great class, everyone.*

Unit 5:
Conflict Resolution

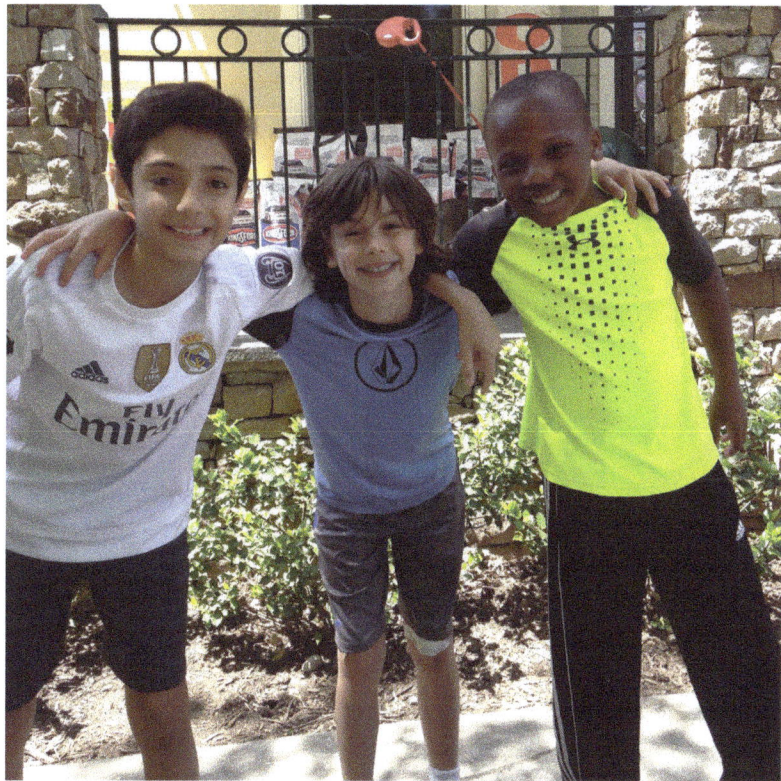

Learn About Conflict with Daisy and Cactus

MINDFULNESS PRACTICE: Color Breaths

OBJECTIVES: Practice mindful breathing and noticing thoughts.

Introduce the word "conflict."

Practice kindness.

PREPARE: A bell or chime

Write the word "conflict" on the board

Your Kindness Pals list

Optional: Brainy the Puppet

Optional: Talking Object

Conflict is a normal part of childhood and of life. Our goal in this unit is to help students integrate all they have been learning about self-awareness, self-regulation, and kindness to solve conflicts peacefully. Many times we tell children to "Calm Down" when they are angry or in a fight without showing them how. Mindfulness practices give children the tools to calm down, to apologize and to use conflict resolution tools like sharing, taking turns, and compromising to help them work things out.

This week students will have another opportunity to integrate all they have learned so far, applying mindfulness and kindness to conflict resolution through acting out a story. We also introduce another new way of practicing mindful breathing called Color Breaths.

Mindfulness Practice

1. **Introduce Color Breaths**

   Say: *Let's think of some new ways to do our Mindful Breathing today! I'm going to say the name of a color and let's see if we can think of ways to do our breathing that match that color.*

Today's color is blue. Can you think of blue things? Remember how we did Wave Breathing? Waves are sort of blue. Who can think of another?

Listen to their ideas and remind everyone to be kind and try other people's ideas. Then when you choose the mindfulness helper you can ask them to choose which idea they want to do again for the "official" Mindful Moment.

2. Mindful Moment

Invite today's Mindfulness Helper (MH) to come to the front of the class to sit next to you on a chair (or next to you on the floor).

Say: *Let's all be happy for _____. (sign language applause)*

Ask the Mindfulness Helper which Blue Breathing they want to do today.

Prompt the MH to say: "Let's get into our mindful bodies. Let's close our eyes or look down. Let's take **three** deep _____ breaths." Everyone will do the Sky Breaths or Blueberry Breaths or whatever they came up with.

Say: *Now take one more deep breath, and listen for the sound of the bell. Try to listen to the whole sound of the bell. Open your eyes or look up when you cannot hear it anymore.*

Ask the MH to ring the bell when the mindful breathing is complete.

Ask the MH to return to their seat.

Conflict Resolution Practice

1. Introduce the word "conflict."

Say: *Today we are going to learn a new word. Has anybody ever heard the word **conflict** before? Does anybody have a guess about what it means?*

Take a few answers.

Remember when we were talking about what happens when we get angry? Well, sometimes when we are angry it is because we have a conflict. A conflict can be any kind of small problem.

Maybe you are having a playdate, and you want to play outside, but your friend wants to play inside. Or maybe you want to play with your brother but he is busy doing his homework.

Conflicts can stay small or they can get bigger.

2. Introduce the story.

Say*: Today we are going to act out a story about two best friends who have a conflict. Their names are Daisy and Cactus. I need two volunteers to act out the story. The volunteers will try to pretend that they are doing what their characters are doing.*

The rest of us are going to be paying close attention. First, I want you to raise your hand if you think you know what their conflict is about. Keep paying attention. Each time you notice one of them flipping their lid, I want you to make the "flipping your lid" gesture. (fingers up, thumb tucked in).

Use Brainy (or your hand) to model the gesture throughout the story.

Choose two actors and ask them to act out the story as you read it. If they feel comfortable, they can repeat their character's lines in addition to pantomiming the actions. Or they can act out the story without speaking.

3. Read the story

<u>Daisy and Cactus </u>by Linda Ryden

Once upon a time there were two friends named Daisy and Cactus. They did everything together. They even had a garden together. They dug holes in the garden together. They planted seeds in their garden together. They waited for the sunshine together. They watered their little plants together. They sang to their little plants together. And together they picked their flowers and vegetables when they were ready. They always worked together and they always shared. Well, almost always….

One day when they were out picking their flowers, Daisy saw the most beautiful rose. It was pink and white and had lots of soft petals. She picked the rose and held it up to her nose to smell it. She said, "Oh how beautiful! This rose makes me so happy!" When Cactus saw that Daisy had the rose, he felt angry. He had been watching that rose all week. He had even given it some extra water. He had planned to pick it and put it in a special vase. And now

Daisy had it. He felt his angry feelings all the way in his belly. His face felt hot, he started breathing faster, and his hands balled up into little fists.

He wanted the rose so badly that he tried to grab it away from Daisy. "Give me my rose!" he shouted. When he grabbed the rose from Daisy he suddenly felt a sharp stinging pain in his fingers. "Ouch! The thorns stung my hand!" Now he was really, really angry so he threw the rose down on the ground and stomped on it with his feet.

When Daisy saw the smashed up rose on the ground she felt angry. "You're so mean, Cactus!" she shouted. "You ruined my beautiful rose!" And she curled up in a ball and cried.

When Cactus saw Daisy crying he felt awful. He really wanted the rose but he didn't want his friend to be so sad. He took five deep breaths until he felt his anger start to get smaller. Then he quickly ran back into the garden and found another rose. This one was yellow and smelled like sunshine. He brought it over to Daisy and said, "I'm sorry I took your rose and smashed it. I was so angry and I flipped my lid."

Daisy took a deep breath as she smelled the yellow rose. "That's okay," she said. "I'm sorry I yelled at you. I guess I flipped my lid too. And I'm sorry you got stung by the thorns. Are you okay?" Daisy wrapped a little piece of green grass around Cactus's finger. "Should we share this yellow rose?" said Cactus. And they went home and put the yellow rose in a beautiful vase.

The End

Choose two more volunteers and act out the story again.

Discuss

1. **Use these questions to guide a discussion.**

   - What was the conflict about?
   - Why was Cactus so angry?
   - How can you tell Cactus has flipped his lid?
   - What did his face look like?
   - What did his body look like?
   - What part of Cactus's brain was in charge?

- Why did Daisy flip her lid?
- Did flipping her lid make her cry?
- Do you ever feel like crying when you are angry?
- Did their conflict get bigger?
- What made it get bigger?
- Did they work out their conflict peacefully? How?

2. Share more generally about conflicts

Ask the class: Have you ever had a conflict with a friend?

Suggest: *Let's share our answers with an elbow partner. Find someone sitting near you and tell him or her about it and then listen to their story.*

I'm going to ring a bell (in 30 seconds or a minute—whatever seems appropriate in the moment) and when you hear the bell, switch to listening to the other person. Let's be mindful that everyone has a partner. Look around and see who needs a partner and if we don't have an even number, see if you can offer to include someone in your group.

You might say, after sharing is over: *So raise your hand if you have ever had a conflict with a friend or someone in your family. Between now and our next time together, try to notice if you have any conflicts. Remember, conflicts are a normal part of life. But we can work out our conflicts peacefully if we try not to flip our lids.*

Kindness Pals

Do the Kindness Pal activity as before.

If there is not enough time for sharing, you can skip that, but be sure to give the students new Kindness Pals.

Closing Words: *Let's have a nice quiet moment with the bell. You can close your eyes or leave them open, but let's sit quietly and listen to the bell. If you want to, you can think about your new Kindness Pal and imagine yourself doing something kind for him or her.*

Ring the bell or chime. *Thanks for a great class, everyone.*

Week 26
The Conflict Escalator

MINDFULNESS PRACTICE: Blooming Breaths

OBJECTIVES:
Practice noticing our thoughts and focusing our attention.

Learn about and use the concept of a Conflict Escalator.

Practice kindness.

PREPARE:
A bell or chime

The Story of Dorothy and Natalie by Linda Ryden

Poster or copies of the Conflict Escalator Worksheet (see Resource Section)

Your Kindness Pals list

Optional: Brainy the Puppet

Optional: Talking Object

The first step to resolving a conflict is recognizing when we are in one and when it is escalating. In this lesson, we will use the concept of a **Conflict Escalator**, developed and named by William Kreidler, to help children understand how and why conflicts get worse. This is a key step in learning how to de-escalate and peacefully resolve conflicts.

Mindfulness Practice

1. Do Blooming Breaths again

Invite today's Mindfulness Helper (MH) to come to the front of the class to sit next to you on a chair (or next to you on the floor).

Say: *Let's all be happy for* _____. *(sign language applause)*

Prompt the MH to say: "Let's get into our mindful bodies. Let's close our eyes or look down. Let's take three deep Blooming Breaths."

Ask the MH to ring the bell when the mindful breathing is complete and return to their seat.

Conflict Resolution Practice

1. **Introduce the Conflict Escalator**

   Draw an escalator on the board. (See Diagram at end of lesson)

   Ask the children to describe what an escalator does.

   Explain that when conflict gets worse, we say that the people involved are going up the Conflict Escalator.

2. **Read the following story to the class.**

   Ask the class to make the "flipping your lid" gesture whenever they notice someone in the story flip their lid. Use Brainy if you like.

   Ask the class to point their finger upwards anytime they notice the conflict get bigger, or go up the conflict escalator.

   The Story of Dorothy and Natalie – Version 1

   Dorothy was unpacking her backpack and her things were spread out on the floor by the cubbies. Natalie was rushing by and tripped over Dorothy's lunch box.

   "Ow!" said Natalie. "Your stuff is everywhere! You made me trip!"

   "No I didn't!" said Dorothy. "You shouldn't have been running!"

   "I wasn't running! I just want to be on time. I don't like to be late, unlike some people," said Natalie.

   "That's mean. You think you're so perfect," said Dorothy.

   "I do not!" said Natalie.

   "Yes you do. (singing) Natalie is perfect, Natalie is perfect…" sang Dorothy.

"You better stop that or I'll stomp all over your stuff!" yelled Natalie.

"You better not!" shouted Dorothy.

Mr. Catapano, their teacher, came into the room and heard all the shouting and commotion. "What's going on here?" he asked.

The girls pointed at each other. "She started it!" they both said.

3. Map the Conflict

Hand out copies of the Conflict Escalator Worksheet. (Found in the Resource Section)

Ask the children to help you diagram the conflict on the conflict escalator on their worksheets.

Read the story again.

4. Discuss.

- What did Dorothy and Natalie say that made them go up the escalator?
- How could they have come down the escalator and solved their problem?
- What do you think happened to them after the teacher came over?
- What could the girls have done differently so that their conflict wouldn't have gone up the Conflict Escalator?

5. Read the second version of the story.

The Story of Dorothy and Natalie – Version 2

Dorothy was unpacking her backpack and her things were spread out on the floor by the cubbies. Natalie was rushing by and tripped over Dorothy's lunch box.

"Ow!" said Natalie. "Your stuff is everywhere! You made me trip!"

Dorothy looked around. Her stuff was everywhere. She didn't like being yelled at but when she took a moment, she realized that it was her fault.

Dorothy took a breath and said, "I'm sorry, Natalie. My stuff is everywhere. Are you okay?"

Natalie smiled and said, "I'm okay. Do you want some help with your stuff?"

"That would be great!" said Dorothy.

6. Discuss.

What did the girls do differently this time**?**

> *NOTE: You can reinforce this lesson by inviting kids to share conflicts they have experienced and asking the class to map them.*

Kindness Pals

Do the Kindness Pal activity as before.

If there is not enough time for sharing, you can skip that, but be sure to give the students new Kindness Pals.

Closing Words: *Let's have a nice quiet moment with the bell. You can close your eyes or leave them open, but let's sit quietly and listen to the bell. If you want to, you can think about your new Kindness Pal and imagine yourself doing something kind for him or her.*

Ring the bell or chime. *Thanks for a great class, everyone.*

The Conflict Escalator

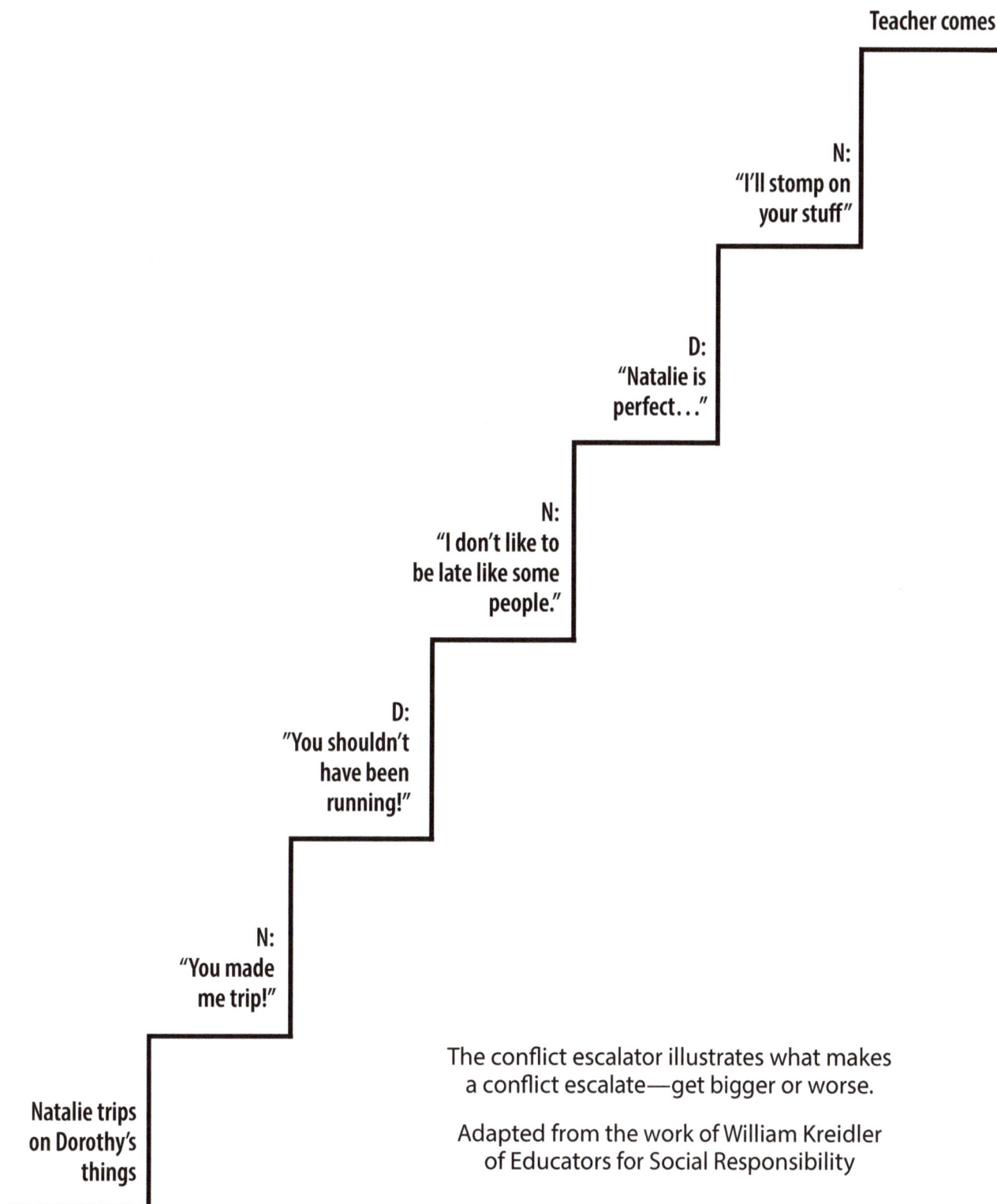

Teacher comes

N:
"I'll stomp on
your stuff"

D:
"Natalie is
perfect…"

N:
"I don't like to
be late like some
people."

D:
"You shouldn't
have been
running!"

N:
"You made
me trip!"

Natalie trips
on Dorothy's
things

The conflict escalator illustrates what makes
a conflict escalate—get bigger or worse.

Adapted from the work of William Kreidler
of Educators for Social Responsibility

The Guinea Pig Conflict

MINDFULNESS PRACTICE: Squeeze and Release

OBJECTIVES: Reinforce the concept of the Conflict Escalator.

Practice kindness.

PREPARE: A bell or chime

The Guinea Pig Conflict by Linda Ryden

Your Kindness Pals list

Poster of or copies of the Conflict Escalator Worksheet (Resource Section)

Optional: Brainy the Puppet

Optional: Talking object

Often when we are in a conflict, our bodies become tight and tense. Our Mindfulness Practice for the day, Squeeze and Release, can really help ease body tension and enable us to calm down so that we can find a good solution to a problem. Today kids will have another chance to practice with the Conflict Escalator. Practicing together in class helps children build a common language and set of tools to use.

Mindfulness Practice

1. Introduce Squeeze and Release

Squeeze and Release is a great practice to do when you are feeling angry or frustrated or any kind of big emotion that makes you feel tight and tense in your body. You exaggerate the feeling of tension in your body and then deliberately try to relax. We've noticed that for some kids it seems easier to try to relax this way. It's also a great way to learn to pay attention to the way that feelings show up in your body.

Say: *Today we're going to learn a mindful breathing practice that can help when your body gets really tight and tense. Have you ever noticed how your body feels when you get angry or frustrated? Do you feel relaxed and loose in your body?*

> **NOTE FROM LINDA:** *I sometimes will demonstrate this by making my body look really relaxed and then say, "Oh I'm so frustrated!" in a really mellow voice. Then I'll make my body look really tight and scrunched up and say, "Hey I'm so relaxed!" in a really tense, tight voice. They usually find it hilarious and it's a good way to help them begin to notice how they feel in their bodies when they are experiencing different emotions.*

It's important to remember and to remind the kids that emotions feel differently for different people. Not everybody feels tight and tense when they get angry. Any way that they feel is fine.

Say: *If you feel tight and tensed up in your body when you get angry you might try something called Squeeze and Release. We'll start with our hands. We're going to breathe in slowly and gently while we are squeezing our hands into little balls. You don't have to do it really hard, but just squeeze it a little. Then when you slowly and gently breathe out you'll try to relax your hands. Let's try it!*

Try a few repetitions. Then move to the shoulders - squeeze them up toward the ears and then gently let them drop down. Squeeze the face and release, then do the stomach muscles, the feet, the whole body, and so on.

Say: *Let's try it for our Mindful Moment!*

2. **Mindful Moment**

    Invite today's Mindfulness Helper (MH) to come to the front of the class to sit next to you on a chair (or next to you on the floor).

    Say: *Let's all be happy for _____.* *(sign language applause)*

    Prompt the MH to say: "Let's get into our mindful bodies. Let's close our eyes or look down. Let's do Squeeze and Release."

    You or the Mindfulness Helper can lead the class through the practice again.

    Ask the MH to ring the bell when the mindful breathing is complete.

    Ask the MH to return to their seat.

Read and Discuss

Marleigh is Mindful

Say: *Today let's see who uses Squeeze and Release in* Marleigh is Mindful. *It's August! Let's hear about August's experience.*

Read the two pages on August and Squeeze and Release.

Ask*:*

- How was August Feeling when he started to do Squeeze and Release? Afterwards?
- How could Squeeze and Release help you?

Conflict Resolution Practice

1. Introduce the lesson.

Draw the Conflict Escalator on the board, or use a copy of the poster in the Resource section.

Review what the Conflict Escalator is. (Lesson 27)

Say*: Today we're going to act out a story about a conflict that happened at school. I will need 5 volunteers. The volunteers will try to pretend that they are doing what their characters are doing.*

2. Choose volunteers to act out the story. Give directions to the class.

Characters: Mr. Cohen, Maurice, Wayne, Lakisha, Bryanna

As before, ask the children to pantomime their character's actions. If they want to repeat their character's lines that's fine. If not, that's fine too.

Say*: Thank you to our volunteers.*

Now everyone else, just like last time, I want you to make the flipping your lid gesture when you notice someone flipping their lid. I also want you to point up when you think the conflict is getting bigger or going up the Conflict Escalator, and point down when you think the conflict is going down the Conflict Escalator.

3. Read and Act out the story.

Read the story and have students act it out.

<u>The Class Guinea Pig</u>

One day Mr. Cohen said to his class, "Look everyone, we have a new class pet. It's a guinea pig!" He held it up for everyone to see. He said, "The four of you get to name it but you have to all agree on the name. Okay?"

Everybody nodded and they got to work.

Maurice said, "I think we should name the guinea pig Luke Skywalker" and he pretended to use a lightsaber.

Lakisha said, "I think we should name the guinea pig Bluebird" and she flew around the room like a bird.

Wayne said, "I think we should name the guinea pig Rainbow," and he pretended to be painting a rainbow.

Bryanna said, "I think we should name the guinea pig Mr. Monkey" and she ran around the room pretending to be a monkey.

Maurice said, "No, those are all terrible names! Luke Skywalker is definitely the best. He has a cool lightsaber."

Lakisha said, "No, Luke Skywalker is a terrible name. He's just a tiny guinea pig, he can't hold a lightsaber."

Wayne said, "Well, he can't fly like a bird either so why would we name him Bluebird?"

Bryanna said, "Monkeys are the coolest so I still think Mr. Monkey is the best name. All of your ideas are bad."

Everybody was feeling angry and beginning to flip their lids. Mr. Cohen came over and said, "So, have you come up with a name yet?"

Freeze the action

4. Discuss.

- What do you think is going to happen if everybody flips their lids?
- Are these kids going up the Conflict Escalator?
- What made their conflict go up the Escalator?

Say: *Let's map their conflict on the Conflict Escalator.*

Write each action or word on the conflict escalator as students suggest them.

Ask: How do you think they should decide what to name the guinea pig?

After they have shared some ideas say: *Okay those are some good ideas. Let's see what happens…*

5. Continue the Story.

Unfreeze the actors and continue the story.

Mr. Cohen said, "So, have you come up with a name yet?" Maurice said sadly, "No, we've just been fighting." Lakisha said, "We all flipped our lids."

Wayne said, "Yeah. We're never going to be able to work out this conflict. "

Bryanna said, "Wait! Why don't we take some deep breaths? That will help us get our lids back on and help us solve our conflict peacefully."

Everybody said, "Great idea!" and they all began to do their Take Five breathing.

Suddenly Lakisha said, "Hey I've got an idea and she ran over to the chalk-board (or whiteboard, or a piece of paper). She wrote on the board MRBLS.

Everybody looked confused. "What is that supposed to be?" asked Maurice. "That's the name!" said Lakisha. "M is for Mr. Monkey, R is for Rainbow, B is for Bluebird and LS is for Luke Skywalker. When you put all of our ideas together you get MRBLS." Wayne said, "What kind of name is MRBLS?" Lakisha said, "If we just add two letters we get the new name." She went to the board and added an A and an E. "Oh I get it," said Bryanna. "Now it spells Marbles!"

And all together they happily shouted, "Welcome to our class, Marbles!"

The End

6. Discuss

- How did the kids calm down so that they could think of a solution?
- How did the kids come up with the new name?

Kindness Pals

Do the Kindness Pal activity as before.

If there is not enough time for sharing, you can skip that, but be sure to give the students new Kindness Pals.

Closing Words: *Let's have a nice quiet moment with the bell. You can close your eyes or leave them open, but let's sit quietly and listen to the bell. If you want to, you can think about your new Kindness Pal and imagine yourself doing something kind for him or her.*

Ring the bell or chime. *Thanks for a great class, everyone.*

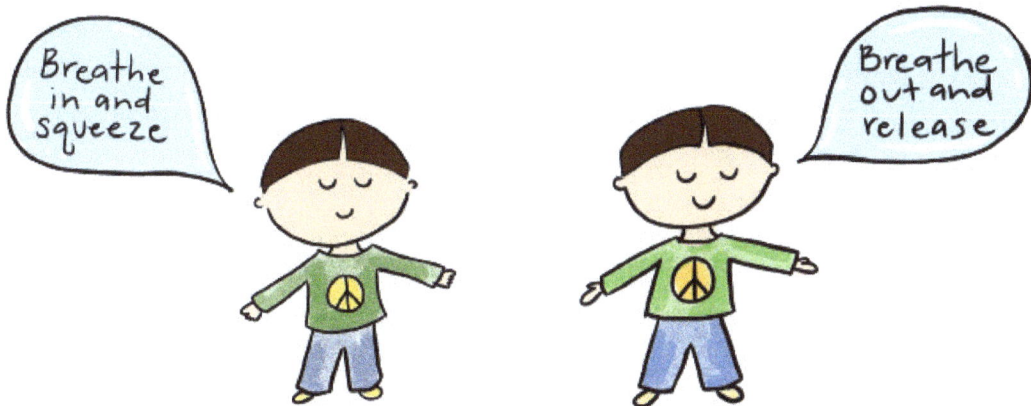

Week 28
Working it Out with Louise and Jack

MINDFULNESS PRACTICE: Squeeze and Release

OBJECTIVES: Learn one method of Conflict Resolution.

Practice kindness.

PREPARE: A bell or chime

The Story of Louise and Jack by Linda Ryden

Jack and Louise Worksheet

Your Kindness Pals list

Optional: Brainy the Puppet

Optional: Talking Object

So far, lessons in this unit have helped students to practice noticing when they are in a conflict, using mindfulness to calm down, and using the tools of apologizing and compromising to solve a conflict. In this lesson, we'll review the relevant brain science and give kids a chance to explore a new conflict resolution tool: sharing.

Mindfulness Practice

1. Squeeze and Release

Say: *Let's try the practice we learned last time called Squeeze and Release. We'll start with our hands. We're going to breathe in slowly and gently while we are squeezing our hands into little balls. You don't have to do it really hard, but just squeeze it a little. Then when you slowly and gently breathe out you'll try to relax your hands. Let's try it!*

Try a few repetitions. Then move to the shoulders - squeeze them up toward the ears and then gently let them drop down. Squeeze the face and release, then do the stomach muscles, the feet, the whole body, etc.

Say: *Let's try it for our Mindful Moment!*

|

2. Mindful Moment

Invite today's Mindfulness Helper (MH) to come to the front of the class to sit next to you on a chair (or next to you on the floor).

Say: *Let's all be happy for _____.* *(sign language applause)*

Prompt the MH to say: "Let's get into our mindful bodies. Let's close our eyes or look down. Let's do Squeeze and Release."

You or the Mindfulness Helper can lead the class through the practice again.

Ask the MH to ring the bell when the mindful breathing is complete.

Ask the MH to return to their seat.

Conflict Resolution Practice

1. Introduce the lesson and review the parts of the brain.

Say: *In the last few lessons we've been learning about conflicts and how they can go up the Conflict Escalator. Today we are going to learn a few ways to bring our conflicts down the Conflict Escalator so we can work them out.*

We're also going to be talking about our brains. Let's review the three parts of the brain we've learned about and what they do. (See lessons 21-23)

Use Brainy to demonstrate.

2. Discuss

Say: *Let's say that you and your brother both want a cookie but there is only one cookie in the cookie jar.*

Use these questions to guide a discussion.

- How would you feel?
- Would you "flip your lid?"
- What would your Amygdala tell you to do?

- What would happen if you listened to your Amygdala?
- What could you do instead (share, eat something else, let your brother have the cookie)?
- Does your Amygdala know how to work out conflicts peacefully?
- What part of your brain knows how to work out conflicts peacefully? (The PFC)
- Do you remember how you can get your PFC in charge again when you have flipped your lid? (take deep breaths)

3. Read and Act out the story.

Say: *I'd like two volunteers to act out a little story.*

Our volunteers are going to pretend to be brother and sister. They are going to act out the story that I am telling using their bodies and their faces. They can repeat their character's lines if they want to.

Everybody else is going to make a Brainy with your hands. One for Louise and one for Jack - just like we did last time. Whenever you notice that Louise is starting to flip her lid, show that with your Brainy. Same for Jack.

Read the following story.

Allow time for the children to act out the activities and emotions you are describing.

The Story of Louise and Jack

Louise and Jack are brother and sister. Usually they get along really well. They like to ride bikes, they like to swim, and they like to read.

Ask the class to come up with other activities Jack and Louise like to do and have the actors act out their ideas.

Today they have been very busy and now they are tired… and hungry.

They walk into their kitchen and reach into the cookie jar and they discover, gasp!, that there is only one cookie left! Oh no!

Louise is very angry and says to Jack, "This is my cookie, let it go!"

Jack says, "No! This is my cookie! You let go!"

They both grab onto the cookie and pull it back and forth between them.

Suddenly, Louise says, "Oh no! We are going up the Conflict Escalator!"

Jack says "You're right. Let's put the cookie down and take some deep breaths."

They both take some nice, deep breaths. Feeling a little calmer, Jack says, "I'm sorry, Louise."

Louise says, "I'm sorry too, Jack. Do you want to share the cookie?" Jack says "Sure!" and splits the cookie in half. Then they happily eat the cookie together.

The End.

3. **Discuss.**

   You might say: *That was a story about how to work out a conflict peacefully.*

   Ask*: Who can tell me what Jack and Louise did to work out their conflict?*

   Take a few answers.

   Say*: That's right, they decided to share the cookie.*

   Ask*: Can you think of any other ways that Jack and Louise could have worked out their conflict?*

4. **Worksheet**

   Activity: Hand out the Louise and Jack worksheets.

   Say: *These pictures are like a comic book version of the story we just acted out. The pictures start when the conflict starts.*

   There are two ways to do this activity:

   1. Have the kids put numbers on each drawing from 1-8 putting them in order as the conflict goes up and down the conflict escalator.

2. Have the kids cut out the pictures and arrange them on their desks in the shape of the escalator going up and down. They can work on their own or with their Kindness Pals.

When they are done then you can go over the answers together.

> *NOTE: Make sure that your students understand why it's so important that the mindful breathing comes **before** the apologizing and working out the conflict.*

Remind them that people don't usually feel like apologizing when they are angry, but once they can calm down people often feel sorry about whatever they did or said that made the conflict escalate.

If you have time, act out the story again with a different solution.

Say: *Next time we will learn about more tools to help us work out conflicts peacefully.*

Kindness Pals

Do the Kindness Pal activity as before.

If there is not enough time for sharing, you can skip that, but be sure to give the students new Kindness Pals.

Closing Words: *Let's have a nice quiet moment with the bell. You can close your eyes or leave them open, but let's sit quietly and listen to the bell. If you want to, you can think about your new Kindness Pal and imagine yourself doing something kind for him or her.*

Ring the bell or chime. *Thanks for a great class, everyone.*

Working it Out with Jahiem and Avi

MINDFULNESS PRACTICE: Gravity Hands

OBJECTIVES: Practice Gravity Hands.

Practice working out conflicts peacefully.

Practice kindness.

PREPARE: A bell or chime

The Story of Jahiem and Avi by Linda Ryden

Jahiem and Avi Worksheet

Your Kindness Pals list and Talking Object

Optional: Brainy the Puppet

Mindfulness Practice

Invite today's Mindfulness Helper (MH) to come to the front of the class to sit next to you on a chair (or next to you on the floor).

Say: *Let's all be happy for _____.* *(sign language applause)*

Prompt the MH to say: "Let's get into our mindful bodies. Let's close our eyes or look down. Let's try Gravity Hands."

Now take a deep breath, and listen for the sound of the bell. Try to listen to the whole sound of the bell. Open your eyes or look down when you cannot hear it anymore.

Ask the MH to ring the bell when the mindful breathing is complete.

Ask the MH to return to their seat.

Conflict Resolution Practice

1. **Review the previous lesson.**

   Say: *Remember last time when we acted out the story about Jack and Louise and the cookie?*

|

Does anybody remember what tool they used to work out their conflict peace-fully? First they calmed down, then they apologized, and then what happened? (They shared the cookie.) Right!

Today we are going to act out another story and learn about some more tools you could use to work out conflicts peacefully.

I'm going to invite two volunteers to act out the story I am telling. Everybody else is going to make a Brainy with your hands. One for Avi and one for Jahiem - just like we did last time. Whenever you notice that Avi is starting to flip his lid, show that with your Brainy. Same for Jahiem.

Ask for two volunteers to act out the story.

2. **Read and Act out the story.**

   The Story of Jahiem and Avi

   Jahiem and Avi are best friends. (They might smile and put their arms around each other's shoulders.)

   They love to play soccer (kick imaginary balls), *draw pictures, and build with Legos.*

   Ask the class to think of other things that Avi and Jahiem like to do together and have the actors act out their ideas.

   Today they are having a playdate and they are so excited!

   Avi says, "Let's go outside. I really want to play soccer!"

   But Jahiem says, "No, I don't feel like being outside. Let's stay inside and draw."

   Avi is really disappointed. He was really looking forward to playing soccer with Jahiem. So, even though he loves drawing, he says, "Drawing is boring! I want to run around. Let's go outside. Only boring people like to draw!"

   Jahiem is really mad now. He doesn't like to be called boring. "Who are you calling boring? You love drawing, Avi. You're being mean."

   Suddenly Avi says, "Wait a minute! We're going up the Conflict Escalator. Oh no!" Jahiem says, "You're right! Let's take some deep breaths so we can calm down a little. I'm starting to flip my lid." Jahiem and Avi take some deep breaths.

Avi says, "That's better. Now I can think again. I'm sorry I said drawing is boring, Jahiem. You know I like drawing with you." Jahiem says, "I know Avi. It's okay. I'm sorry I said you were being mean."

Freeze the action.

3. **Discuss.**

- Why was Avi so mad?
- Why does he say drawing is boring even though he likes drawing? (He's flipped his lid.)
- Have you ever felt this way?

Give the class a chance to consider resolutions to this conflict. Ask:

- Can anybody think of a peaceful way for the boys to work out this conflict?
- Will the solution we saw last time—sharing—work here? Why or why not?
- What else could they do? (They will probably suggest taking turns or doing some combination of drawing and soccer, or perhaps flipping a coin.)

   After you hear their ideas, turn back to the story by saying: *Okay, those are great ideas! Let's find out how Avi and Jahiem solved their problem.*

4. **Continue the story.**

   Direct the actors to "Unfreeze." Read the following:

   Jahiem says, "Hey Avi, I've got an idea. Why don't we play soccer for half an hour and then come inside and draw for half an hour?"

   Avi says, "That's a great idea! We can take turns. Thanks Jahiem!"

   Jahiem says "No problem! Let's go!" (They kick around the ball around a little.)

   Half an hour later… (They pretend to draw.)

   The End

5. Repeat the story.

Say: *Okay, so who can tell me what tool Jahiem and Avi used to work out their conflict? That's right, they decided to take turns. Taking turns is a great way to work out many conflicts. But there are lots of ways to work out conflicts.*

Let's act out the story again and this time let's see if we can think of a different tool to use to work out the conflict.

Act out the story again, choosing two new kids.

This time, solve the problem in a different way. Feel free to change the activities they want to do, the names, and so on to reflect the needs and interests of your class.

Next time Jahiem could offer to let Avi choose what they do or just "be kind". Maybe they could decide to draw pictures about soccer, or they could compromise and do something else entirely like watch a movie. Let the kids be creative but remind them that we want to find a solution that makes both people feel okay.

Make sure that someone says: "We're going up the Conflict Escalator." That serves as a reset button for the conflict.

6. Worksheet

Do the worksheet activity the same way as in the previous lesson. This time the 8th square is left blank. Ask the kids to draw a picture of a different solution to the conflict. They can work with a partner or on their own.

Go over their answers as well as their ideas for solutions to the conflict.

Kindness Pals

Do the Kindness Pal activity as before.

If there is not enough time for sharing, you can skip that, but be sure to give the students new Kindness Pals.

Closing Words: *Let's have a nice quiet moment with the bell. You can close your eyes or leave them open, but let's sit quietly and listen to the bell.   If you want to, you can think about your new Kindness Pal and imagine yourself doing something kind for him or her.*

Ring the bell or chime. *Thanks for a great class, everyone6*

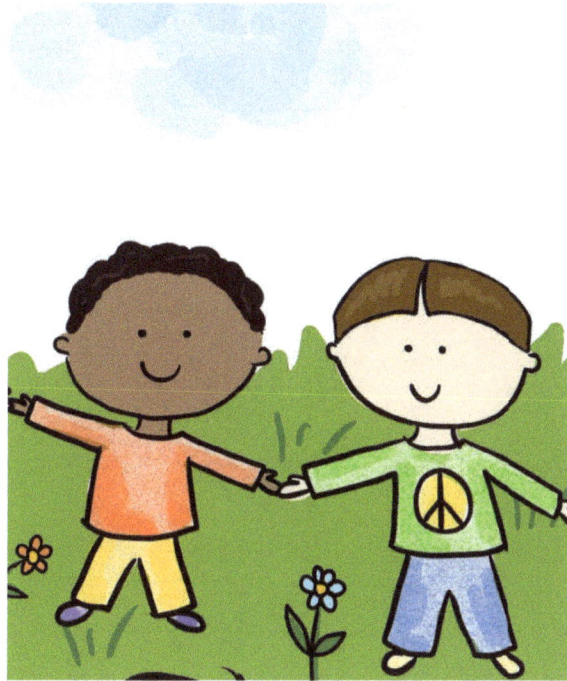

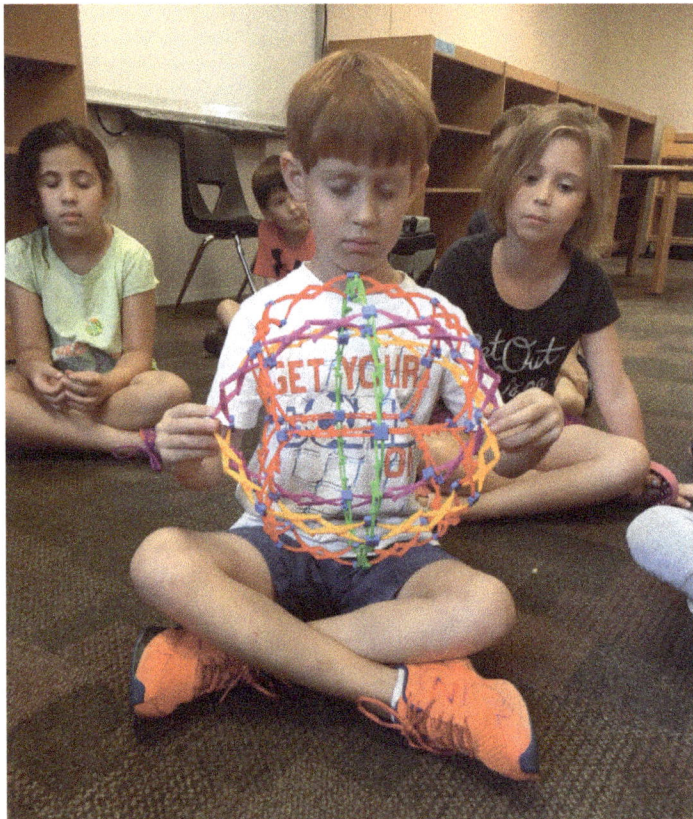

UNIT 6:
Kindness

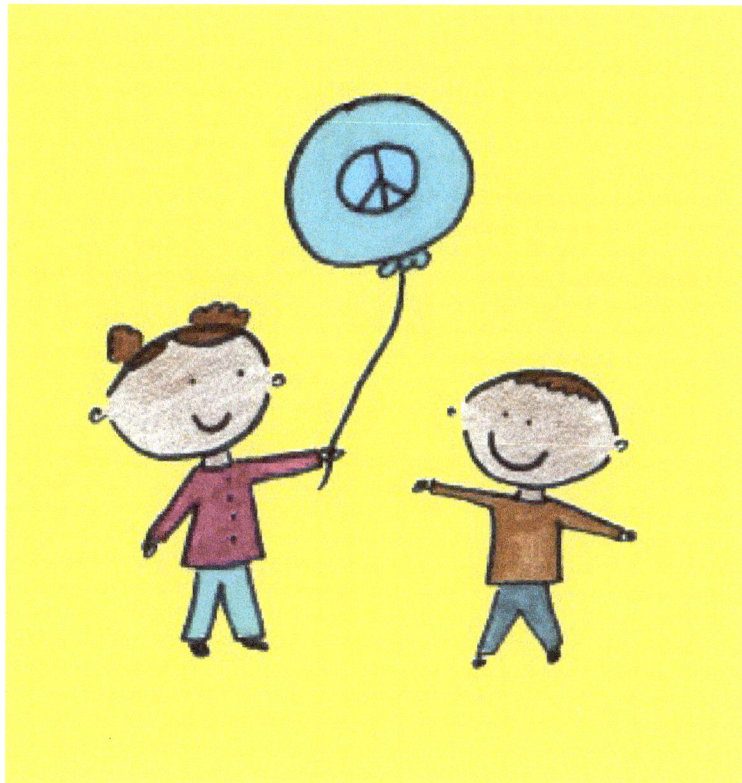

Henry is Kind

MINDFULNESS PRACTICE: Heartfulness

OBJECTIVES: Help the children get into the habit of doing kind things.

Notice the good feelings that come from showing kindness to others.

Practice Heartfulness.

PREPARE: A bell or chime

Henry is Kind by Linda Ryden

Chart paper for making an Anchor Chart

Sticky notes with hearts drawn on them

Kind to Me Worksheet

Your Kindness Pals list and Talking Object

Here we are in the last unit of the Curriculum. We end with three lessons that focus on one of the most important things we can think of to share with a child: kindness. Throughout the year your students have been practicing being kind through Kindness Pals and building classroom community. Today, they will have another chance to practice heartfulness and read and talk about the book *Henry is Kind*.

Mindfulness Practice

Say: *Today we are going to do Heartfulness. Do you remember doing this before? This just means that we are going to be thinking about a person and sending them kind thoughts.*

We aren't going to be making them a card or talking to them. We are going to be thinking kind thoughts about them in our minds. Let's start out as we always do with our Mindfulness Helper and then I'll remind you about how it works.

Invite today's Mindfulness Helper (MH) to come to the front of the class to sit next to you on a chair (or next to you on the floor).

Say: *Let's all be happy for* _____. *(sign language applause)*

Say: *Today we are going to practice Heartfulness.*

Prompt the MH to say: "Let's get into our mindful bodies. Let's close our eyes or look down. Let's take three deep breaths."

Say: *I'd like you to think about someone who makes you happy.* **Choose someone you see every day** *at home or at school. You might choose someone in your family, a friend, teacher, even a pet. Just choose someone and try to picture that person happy and smiling. Picture them doing something that makes them happy. Try to notice how you feel when you think about this person.*

Now, if you'd like to, fill your heart up with kindness and repeat these words in your mind while you think about this person. I will say the words out loud and you may think them in your mind or whisper them quietly.

May you be happy. **Wait a moment to give them time to repeat the words.**

May you be healthy. **Wait a moment.**

May you be peaceful. **Wait a moment.**

Take a moment to notice how you feel. Any way that you feel is fine, even if you feel nothing. Just try to notice it.

Now take a deep breath, and listen for the sound of the bell. Try to listen to the whole sound of the bell. Open your eyes or look up when you cannot hear it anymore.

Ask the MH to ring the bell when the mindful breathing is complete.

Ask the MH to return to their seat.

Invite the students to share whom they were thinking about or how it felt.

Kindness Practice

1. **Introduce the lesson.**

   Say: *Today we are going to be thinking about how we are kind to other people and how other people are kind to us. We're going to start by reading a story.*

2. **Read the book <u>Henry is Kind</u>**

This is the story of a boy who doesn't think he is kind to other people. Other kids in his class point out all of the ways that he has been kind that he doesn't even remember.

3. **Activity: Make an Anchor Chart**

Draw a big heart on the white board or on chart paper and draw hearts on a bunch of sticky notes. Every time someone in the book does something kind, ask the children to raise their hands and then choose someone to come up and put a sticky note on the big heart. At the end of the story try to remember what the hearts stand for and count up all of the acts of kindness.

4. **Activity: Kind To Me Worksheet**

Have the students think of examples of acts of kindness that people have done for them or for others. Then have them draw about a time that someone was kind to them on the *Kind To Me* Worksheet.

5. **Optional Activity - Kindness Box**

Make a box to keep in your classroom called the Kindness Box. Leave little pieces of paper near the box so that when kids "catch" other people being kind they can write it down and put it in the box. Once in a while you can open the box and read about all of the acts of kindness!

Kindness Pals

Do the Kindness Pals activity as before.

Closing Words: *Let's have a nice quiet moment with the bell. You can close your eyes or leave them open, but let's sit quietly and listen to the bell. If you want to, you can think about your new Kindness Pal and imagine yourself doing something kind for him or her.*

Ring the bell or chime. *Thanks for a great class, everyone.*

Week 31
Gratitude Cards

MINDFULNESS PRACTICE: Heartfulness

OBJECTIVES:

Practice mindful gratitude.

Encourage the children to appreciate the kindness of the people around them and to practice expressing that gratitude.

PREPARE:

A bell or chime

Enough paper folded in half like a card for all of the school staff you will thank, crayons or markers

Index cards with the names and jobs of school staff written on them, making sure to include office staff, custodians, school resource officers, and so on

Your Kindness Pals list and Talking Object

In this lesson, students will make gratitude cards for school staff and, if possible, hand deliver them. This is an opportunity for children to express their thanks in a kind way to all of those who have made their school year possible.

NOTE FROM LINDA: *I'll never forget the looks on two of my students' faces after they delivered their gratitude cards to the cafeteria manager. She is a little crusty and some kids are afraid of her. With huge smiles on their faces they told me and the rest of the class how much she had smiled, and even cried a little when she got the cards and that she came around from behind the counter to give them both big hugs. These boys hadn't been that excited about the project but now they wanted to make more and more cards to spread the love!*

Mindfulness Practice

Say: *This is our second to last Peace of Mind class for this year. We have learned so many different ways to practice mindfulness - at least 15! And that's not even counting all of the ones you created yourselves. Let's see how many we can remember.*

Make a list on the board or chart paper of all the mindfulness practices they can remember (with some prompting, of course!). Your list could include;

Mindful listening, Animal Breaths, Tummy Breathing, Take Five, Mindful Seeing, Find the Rainbow, Heartfulness, Mindful Movements, Wave Breaths, Nature Breaths, Gratitude Cups, Flower Breaths, Bubble Breaths, Candle Breaths, and Straw Breaths

Review all of the practices (show the pictures from Marleigh is Mindful if you'd like). Then ask the Mindfulness Helper to choose which one you will do for your Mindful Moment today.

Invite today's Mindfulness Helper (MH) to come to the front of the class to sit next to you on a chair (or next to you on the floor).

Say: *Let's all be happy for _____.* (sign language applause)

Prompt the MH to say: "Let's get into our mindful bodies. Let's close our eyes or look down. Let's do _____."

Now take a deep breath, and listen for the sound of the bell. Try to listen to the whole sound of the bell. Open your eyes or look up when you cannot hear it anymore.

Ask the MH to ring the bell when the mindful breathing is complete.

Ask the MH to return to their seat.

Gratitude Practice

1. **Introduce the lesson.**

   You might say:

Today we are going to be saying thank you to some important people in our lives. I know that many of you have made birthday cards for your parents or maybe a thank you card for a favorite teacher.

But have you ever said thank you to our custodians? Or the front-office staff? Or the nice people who make our lunches in the cafeteria? Well, here's your chance!

Today we are going to show our thanks to these special people who keep our school running. I am going to give you an index card with somebody's name on it, and I'd like you to make them a thank you card to express our gratitude for all of their hard work.

2. Create cards.

Distribute supplies: paper and crayons and markers.

Give out index cards with names of staff, custodians, and so on. If possible, include pictures of each person.

Collect the cards when students are finished.

> *NOTE: Some kids are going to be really insistent about who they want to make a card for. Classroom teachers receive lots of thanks and kids always want to make a card for their favorite teacher from last year. Try to encourage them to spread that love, even to someone they don't know.*

You might tell the kids that they can make a card for anyone they want as long as they first make one for the person on their index card. Remind them how important it is for everyone to get a card—like on Valentine's Day when we make cards for everyone, not just the kids we like the best. If it's possible, have the children hand-deliver the cards.

Kindness Pals

Do the Kindness Pals activity as before.

Closing Words: *Let's have a nice quiet moment with the bell. You can close your eyes or leave them open, but let's sit quietly and listen to the bell. If you want to, you can think about your new Kindness Pal and imagine yourself doing something kind for him or her.*

Ring the bell or chime. *Thanks for a great class, everyone.*

Week 32
The Kindness Chain

MINDFULNESS PRACTICE: Heartfulness

OBJECTIVES:
Practice mindful breathing.

Illustrate the power of words to start a chain of kindness.

Make a kindness chain.

Practice kindness.

PREPARE:
A bell or chime

Your Kindness Pals list and Talking Object

This is our last class! Congratulations for bringing your students through another year. What a wonderful thing you have done! We hope that Peace of Mind has been of help in building a strong and positive classroom community. Today we are focusing on expressing kindness and appreciation for ourselves and each other. We hope you enjoy this final class together!

Mindfulness Practice

Say: *For our final class let's do Heartfulness. It can feel really good to think about each other and share some love and kindness. The Mindfulness Helper can choose how we are going to take our three deep breaths and then I will lead us through the Heartfulness practice.*

Invite today's Mindfulness Helper (MH) to come to the front of the class to sit next to you on a chair (or next to you on the floor).

Say: *Let's all be happy for _____. (sign language applause)*

Prompt the MH to say: "Let's get into our mindful bodies. Let's close our eyes or look down. Let's take three deep _____ breaths."

Say: *Now let's start by thinking some kind thoughts for ourselves. Think about how hard you worked this year, all of the kind things you did in our classroom, all of the things that you learned and how much you have grown. You can give yourself a little hug if you want to.*

Now I'll say the words out loud and you can quietly whisper them or think them in your mind.

May I be happy. Wait

May I be healthy and strong. Wait

May I be peaceful. Wait

Now let's send some kindness to one of your classmates. Just choose one person in the class and hold a picture of them in your mind and heart.

May you be happy. Wait

May you be healthy and strong. Wait

May you be peaceful. Wait

Now let's send some kindness to the whole class. Think of all of us. All of us who have spent this year learning and growing together.

May we all be happy. Wait

May we all be healthy and strong. Wait

May we all be peaceful. Wait

Say: *Now take one more deep breath, and listen for the sound of the bell. Try to listen to the whole sound of the bell. Open your eyes or look up when you cannot hear it anymore.*

Ask the MH to ring the bell and return to their seat.

Discuss

Invite children to share what they felt.

Kindness Practice

1. **Introduce the Kindness Chain.**

   Say: *Today we are going to be using our words to make people feel good.*

   Today we are going to make a Kindness Chain. The first step is to gather into a circle.

We are going to go around the circle and I'd like you to say something kind about the person sitting to your right. For example, I might say, "Cheryl, you are an awesome friend."

Cheryl might say "Thanks!" and then turn to the person on her right and say, "Harry, you are really good at building things."

And we'll go around the circle like that. Every once in a while when we play this game somebody's mind goes blank and they can't think of anything to say— even if they are sitting next to their best friend! If that happens to you, don't worry. Just say, "I need some help," and I will choose a volunteer to say something kind about that person. Then we'll continue going around the circle.

When we're done, we'll go around the circle in the other direction.

This is a chance to use the power of our words to make people feel really good so let's try hard to take it seriously and make sure that everybody feels good. Ready to start?"

2. Share and reflect.

Ask the children to share what it felt like to give and receive these compliments and what it feels like to use the power of your words for good.

3. Optional Activity - Make a Paper Kindness Chain

Give each child a strip of construction paper and have them write something kind about someone in the class on it. Then put the whole chain together and hang it in the classroom.

Kindness Pals

Do Kindness Pals as before, but do not give out new pals.

Closing words: *This is our last class together, so I will not be handing out new kindness pals today.*

I hope that you enjoyed learning more about mindfulness, kindness, and how to work out our conflicts peacefully. The world needs lots of kind, mindful people. Now you have some tools to help you go out into the world and make it a more peaceful place. I hope you will!

Resources

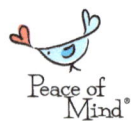

Program Extensions

Consider moving the lessons of *Peace of Mind* beyond the classroom with one or more of these Program extensions. Each offers opportunities for students to hone their new mindfulness skills, to practice kindness, and to use the common language and tools they are learning to resolve conflicts.

Daily Mindful Moments

Peace of Mind is designed as a weekly curriculum. However, if you have the time and desire to make *Peace of Mind* a part of your classroom every day, we salute you! Daily Mindful Moments are a great way for your students to practice the skills that they are learning weekly in *Peace of Mind* class, and to enjoy a moment of calm and quiet before beginning a new activity. You might institute a Mindful Moment at the beginning of the day, after recess, or before math, for example.

You may want to make "Mindfulness Helper" a weekly job in your classroom and have that student lead the Daily Mindful Moment. You may decide to lead the Daily Mindful Moment yourself at the beginning to set the tone and expectations, and then transition to a student-led practice. Either way is fine.

You can experiment with the duration of the quiet moment. Some classes will have no problem with two minutes and will quickly graduate to more; some classes will be better off with one minute or less to start. Choose a short mindfulness practice to follow, including the Mindfulness Helper, or do it your own way.

Once you get into the habit, Mindful Moments will be beneficial to both you and your students.

Peace Club

At Lafayette Elementary School, where the Peace of Mind Program was developed, Peace Club is a lunch and recess program for students who need a smaller alternative to the cafeteria and the playground. It can be a mixed-age group of anywhere from 20-50 students. Peace Club is meant to be a comfortable option for kids who sometimes struggle with their social skills or with being in a large group. It is also popular among kids who like to make a difference and who make a commitment to helping everyone feel welcome and respected.

At Lafayette, for example, children on the autism spectrum and with other diagnoses often have Peace Club specifically written into their educational plans because Peace Club provides some structured play as well as informal group counseling during the hour.

Peace Club requires all students who come to make a promise to treat everyone else with kindness and respect, and to make sure that conflicts are worked out peacefully and everyone is included. Fourth and fifth graders might serve as special helpers. These are kids who make an extra commitment to seek out those who have a harder time jumping in and include them in games, and who help others work out conflicts peacefully.

Peace Heroes

Peace Heroes is a way to recognize children who make an extra effort to be kind. One way to do this is to have a box somewhere in the school where kids or adults can write a note recognizing another student for an act of kindness. The names can be posted on a bulletin board somewhere in the school. Once a month some of the names can be read on school-wide announcements.

Linkages to Other Programs

The concepts underlying the *Peace of Mind* program can be adapted to work with other programs like Positive Behavioral Intervention and Supports (PBIS) and Responsive Classroom. School-wide expectations can be expressed in "mindful" language—for example "Speak Mindfully, Act Mindfully, Move Mindfully." Most of the things that we are expecting the children to do at school fall into these three categories. Children can be encouraged to "move mindfully" in the hallways, instead of saying "No running!" or to "speak mindfully" instead of "don't blurt out," or to "act mindfully" instead of "be responsible." This subtle shift in language can help children understand the reasons for our rules and make them more likely to follow them.

Reproducible Materials

In this section you will find the following reproducible worksheets for your class.

All weeks: Kindness Pals Template

Week 1: My Kindness Pal Worksheet

Week 2: Animal Breaths Worksheet

Week 4: Take Five Breathing Worksheet

Week 5: Find the Rainbow Worksheet

Week 7: Heartfulness Worksheet

Week 9: Create Your Own Way of Breathing Worksheet

Week 10: I Am Grateful For Worksheet

Week 13: Gratefuls Box Worksheet (optional)

Week 17: Finding Your Feelings Worksheet

Week 18: Commonalities Worksheet

Week 19: Visualization Worksheet

For Unit 4: Diagram of Three Parts of the Brain

Week 21: Amygdala Worksheet

For Unit 5: The Conflict Escalator Worksheet

Week 28: Jack and Louise Worksheet

Week 29: Jahiem and Avi Worksheet

Week 30: Kind To Me Worksheet

|

Kindness Pals

for the week of _____

	Student	Student
1.		
2.		
3.		
4.		
5.		
6.		
7.		
8.		
9.		
10.		
11.		
12.		
13.		
14.		
15.		

My Kindness Pal Worksheet

Here are some kind acts I can do for my pal. Circle all those you might choose.

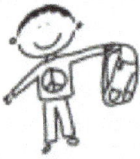

Get backpack

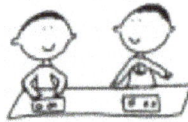

Eat lunch together

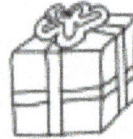

Small gift

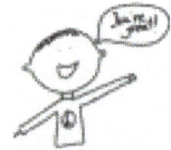

Compliment

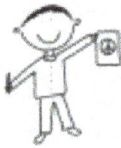

Draw a picture

Stack chair

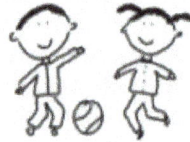

Play at recess

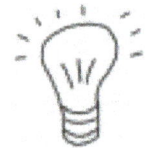

Another idea

Make up your own Animal Breath!

My Animal Breath is called: _____

Breathe slowly in and out.

Your Name: _____

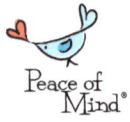

Calm Down with Take Five Breathing

Breathe in and out as you trace your hand.

My Name: _____

Find the Rainbow!

When you feel angry or upset you can find something around you for each color of the rainbow. It can help you to calm down. Find something for each color and draw it in the square!

I found something red:	I found something orange:	I found something yellow:
I found something green:	I found something blue:	I found something purple:

My Name: _____

Week 7
Heartfulness

I sent my kind thoughts to...

May you be happy.
May you be healthy and strong.
May you be peaceful.

My Name: _____

|

Week 9
Create Your Own Way of Breathing

My breathing movement is called_____

My Name: _____

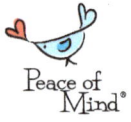

I am Grateful for...

Draw a picture here of something you are grateful for.

\

My Name: _____

Gratefuls Box

What will you put in your Gratefuls Box today?

MY GRATEFULS BOX

My Name: _____

Finding Your Feelings

Draw a picture of yourself and point to where you could feel happiness, anger, sadness, or surprise.

My Name: _____

Week 18
Commonalities

What do we have in common?

What is your favorite:

Animal?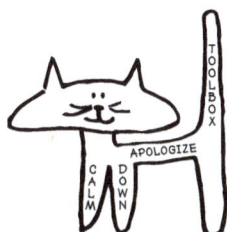

Part of the school day?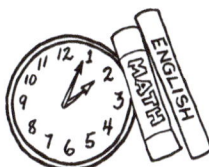

Ice Cream Flavor?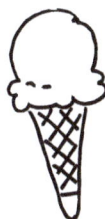

Candy?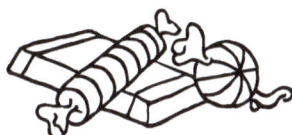

TV show?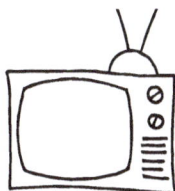

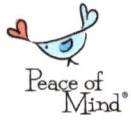

Draw a Picture of Your Park

My Name: _____

Diagram of Three Parts of the Brain

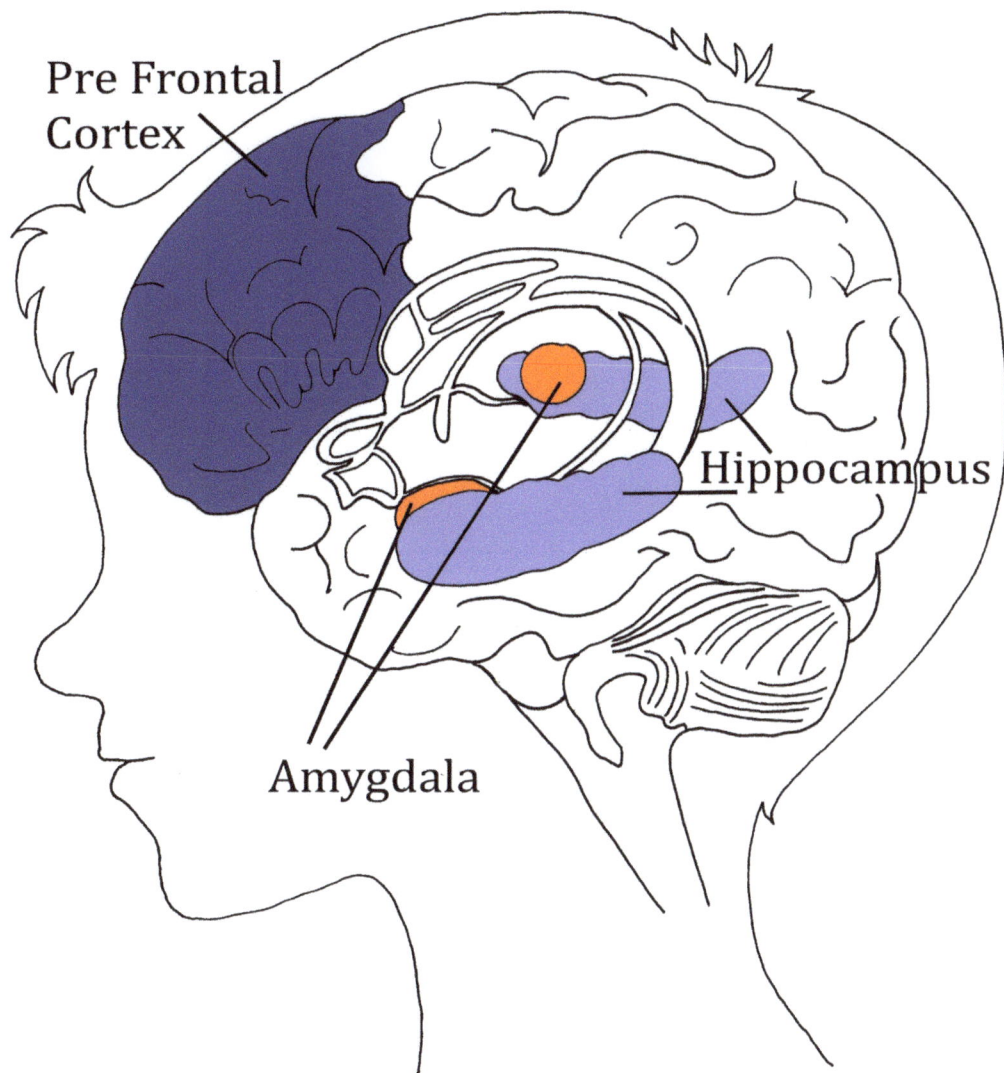

Pre Frontal Cortex

Hippocampus

Amygdala

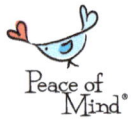

Amygdala

Can you think of a time when "Amy" tried to help you?

My Name: _____

The Conflict Escalator

BIG
TROUBLE!

small
problem

Louise and Jack

The Cookie Conflict

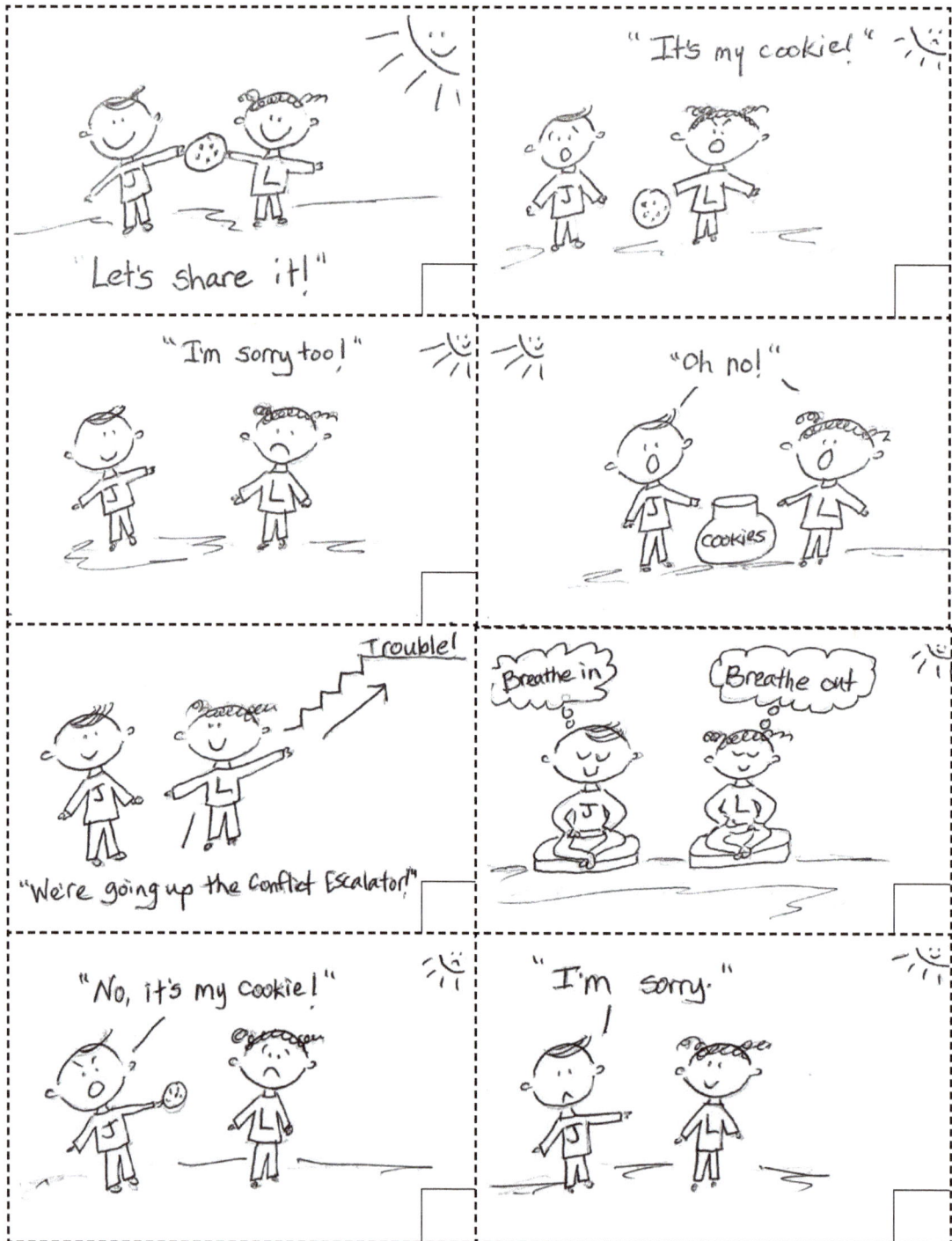

Name_____

Week 29

Jahiem and Avi

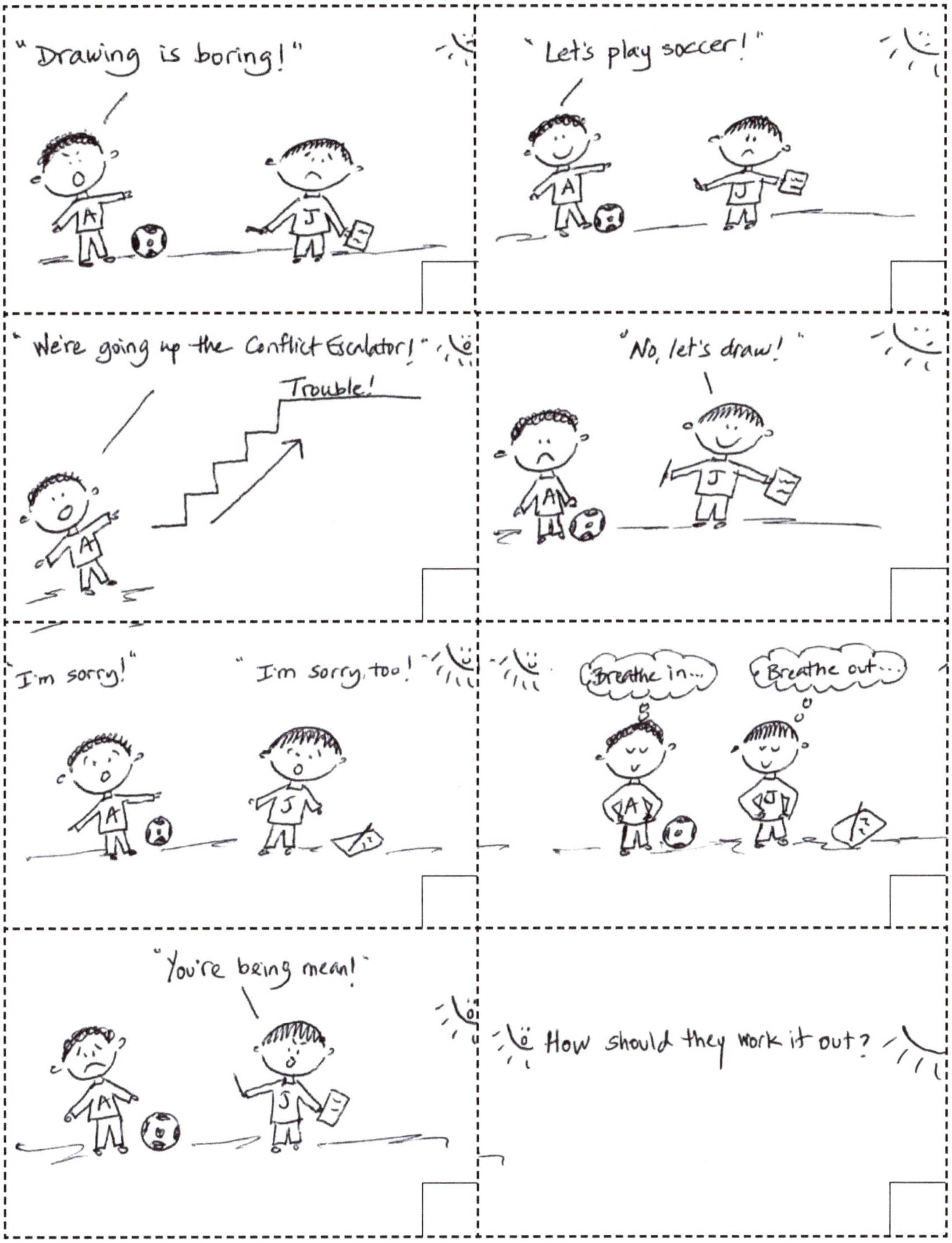

Name____

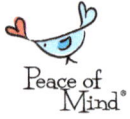

Week 30
People are Kind to Me!

Draw a picture of a time when someone was kind to you

My Name: _____

Resources to Support You and Your Teaching

Here are just a few of the many books, apps, podcasts and websites we've found helpful. Each of them will point you to other resources. Enjoy!

Your Own Mindfulness Practice

Apps

Headspace.com
Ten Percent Happier App and Podcast
Calm, especially Jeff Warren's Daily Trip and How To Meditate Series

Online Mindfulness Courses

Mindful Schools Courses for Educators
https://www.mindfulschools.org/

Elements of Meditation with Jeff Warren
https://jeffwarren.THiNKific.com/courses/

Good Reads

You Belong: A Call for Connection by Sebene Selassie

The Mindful Athlete by George Mumford

Ten Percent Happier and Meditation for Fidgety Skeptics by Dan Harris and Jeff Warren

Hardwiring Happiness by Dr. Rick Hanson

Teaching Mindfulness

Mindfulness for teachers: Simple skills for peace and productivity in the classroom by Patricia Jennings

The Way of Mindful Education: Cultivating Well-being in Teachers and Students by Daniel Rechtschaffen & Jon Kabat-Zinn PhD

Compassion and Gratitude

Real Love by Sharon Salzberg

Center for the Greater Good at U.C. Berkeley
https://greatergood.berkeley.edu/

Center for Healthy Minds at the U. of Wisconsin
https://centerhealthyminds.org/

Brain Science

Daniel Siegel's Brain Talk Video (YouTube)
http://www.drdansiegel.com/resources/everyday_mindsight_tools/

Trauma Sensitive Teaching

Jennings, P. A. (2019). *The Trauma-Sensitive Classroom: Building Resilience with Compassionate Teaching*. New York: W.W. Norton & Company.

Treleaven, David (2018). *Trauma-Sensitive Mindfulness: Practices for Safe and Transformative Healing.* New York: W. W. Norton & Company.

Teaching for Social Justice

Starting in Grade 3, lessons in our Peace of Mind Curriculum Series include the application of Mindfulness-based SEL to social justice topics like identity, discrmination, bias and standing up to injustice. Though your students won't receive these lessons for another year or two, you might like to learn more about some of these topics now as a way to support your teaching in general.

Here are some options:

Why We Can't Afford Whitewashed Social and Emotional Learning by Dr. Dena Simmons
http://www.ascd.org/publications/newsletters/education_update/apr19/vol61/num04/Why_We_Can't_Afford_Whitewashed_Social-Emotional_Learning.aspx

Racial Healing Allies
https://www.ticiess.com/racial-healing-allies

AntiRacist Table
theantiracisttable.com

LiberatED
denasimmons.com

Learning for Justice
learningforjustice.org

Center for AntiRacist Education
antiracistfuture.org

Bibliography

Bradshaw, C. P. (2015). Translating research to practice in bullying prevention. American Psychologist, 70 (4), 322-332.

Breeding, K., & Harrison, J. (2007). *Connected and Respected: Lessons from the Resolving Conflict Creatively Program.* Cambridge, Mass.: Educators for Social Responsibility.

Durlak, J. A., Weissberg, R. P., Dymnicki, A. B., Taylor, R. D. & Schellinger, K. B. (2011). The impact of enhancing students' social and emotional learning: A meta-analysis of school-based universal interventions. Child Development, 82(1): 405–432.

Greater Good Science Center, White Paper prepared for the John Templeton Foundation, retrieved from: https://ggsc.berkeley.edu/images/uploads/GGSC-JTF_White_Paper-Gratitude-FINAL.pdf?_ga=2.243809989.1952658949.1625427932-835142985.1625427932 on July 6. 2021.

Hanson, R. (2015). *Hardwiring Happiness.* Random House USA.

Jennings, P. (2015). *Mindfulness for teachers: Simple skills for peace and productivity in the classroom.* The Norton Series on the Social Neuroscience of Education.

Jennings, P. A. (2019). *The Trauma-Sensitive Classroom: Building Resilience with Compassionate Teaching.* New York: W.W. Norton & Company.

Lantieri, Linda. "How SEL and Mindfulness Can Work Together." Greater Good. April 7, 2015. Accessed September 28, 2015. http://greatergood.berkeley.edu/article/item/how_social_emotional_learning_and_mindfulness_can_work_together.

Learning Heroes, *Developing Life Skills in Children: A Road Map for Communicating with Parents*, https://bealearninghero.org/parent-mindsets/ September 2018

O'Brennan, L., & Bradshaw, C. (2013). School Climate: A Research Brief. A report prepared for the National Education Association, Washington, DC.

Rechtschaffen, D., & Kabat-Zinn PhD, J. (2014). *The Way of Mindful Education: Cultivating Well-being in Teachers and Students.* Norton Books in Education. Schonert-Reichl, K. A., & Lawlor, M. S. (2010). The effects of a mindfulness-based education program on pre-and early adolescents' well-being and social and emotional competence. *Mindfulness, 1*(3), 137-151.

Salberg, Sharon (2018), *Real Love.* Flatiron Books; Reprint edition

Schonert-Reichl, K. A., Oberle, E., Lawlor, M. S., Abbott, D., Thomson, K., Oberlander, T. F., & Diamond, A. (2015). Enhancing cognitive and social–emotional development through a simple-to-administer mindfulness-based school program for elementary school children: A randomized controlled trial. *Developmental Psychology, 51*(1), 52-66.

Selassie, Sebene (2020), *You Belong: A Call for Connection* HarperOne

Seppala, E., Simon-Thomas, E., Brown, S. L., Worline, M. C., Cameron, C. D., & Doty, J. R. (2017). *The Oxford Handbook of Compassion Science*. New York, NY: Oxford University Press.

Siegel, D. J., & Bryson, T. P. (2012). *The Whole-Brain Child*. London: Constable & Robinson.

Simmons, Dena (2019), *Why We Can't Afford Whitewashed Social-Emotional Learning* Retrieved from http://www.ascd.org/publications/newsletters/education_update/apr19/vol61/num04

Srinivasan, M. (2014). *Teach, Breathe, Learn: Mindfulness in and out of the Classroom*. Berkeley, CA: Parallax Press.

Treleaven, David (2018). *Trauma-Sensitive Mindfulness: Practices for Safe and Transformative Healing*. New York: W. W. Norton & Company.

Weare, K. (2013). Developing mindfulness with children and young people: A review of the evidence and policy context. *Journal of Children's Services, 8(*2), 141-153.

Zoogman, S., Goldberg, S.B., Hoyt, W.T., & Miller, L. (2015). Mindfulness interventions with youth: A meta-analysis. *Mindfulness, 6*, 290 - 302.

Zenner, C., Hermleben-Kurz, S., & Walach, H. (2014). Mindfulness-based interventions in schools: A systematic review and meta-analysis. *Frontiers in Psychology, 5*, article 603.

Credits

Hand Model of the Brain. Lessons 20-24: "Everyday Mindsight Tools." Dr. Dan Siegel. March 17, 2011. Accessed September 28, 2015. http://www.drdansiegel.com/resources/everyday_mindsight_tools/

The Conflict Escalator. Lessons 26-29: Kreidler, William J. *Teaching Conflict Resolution through Children's Literature*. New York: Scholastic Professional Books, 1994

Blooming Breaths. Lessons 23 and 26. Alexis Larson, 2021.

Acknowledgements

Appreciation

Linda's students have been our greatest teachers, our inspiration, and our joy. Each one of the more than 1,000 children Linda has worked with at Lafayette Elementary School in Washington, D.C. has taught us something important, and some have left lasting imprints on our hearts. These children, some of who are in college now, fill us with hope that they will create a more peaceful world than the one they were born into.

We owe a huge debt of gratitude to the wonderful teachers Lafayette Elementary and all of the other Washington DC area Schools who have welcomed and supported the *Peace of Mind* Program from its earliest days. Leaders Liz Whisnant, Megan Vroman and Jordan Love, especially, have gone above and beyond.

Lafayette's amazing School Counselor Jillian Diesner took on the challenge of adapting the *Peace of Mind* curriculum to our youngest students and has contributed so much of her expertise and creativity to expand *Peace of Mind* in wonderful new ways.

In this testing-focused culture it takes courage to set aside time in the school day for something that can't be easily quantified. Many thanks to Lafayette Principal Dr. Carrie Broquard for her enthusiastic support for the *Peace of Mind* program. Thanks to her leadership and willingness to go out on a limb, *Peace of Mind* has grown into an effective model program.

Peace of Mind would not have been possible without the generous financial support of the Lafayette Home and School Association. Many thanks to all members, past and present, for supporting the program over the years, and for making our children's social emotional development a priority.

We are grateful to the many people whose work inspires and informs the *Peace of Mind Program*. So much of what is offered in these pages is inspired by the work of these wonderful teachers: Jeff Warren, Dan Harris, Rick Hanson, Sharon Salzberg, Oren Jay Sofer, Jay Michelson, and Sebene Selassie.

Our nonprofit organization, Peace of Mind Inc, is guided and sustained by an extraordinary Board of Directors. Enormous thanks to Liz Whisnant, Darrel Jodrey, Chapin Springer, Dr. Elizabeth Hoffman, and Subrat Biswal for all that you give and have given. Thanks, too, to our Advisors whose input has been invaluable: Rie Odsbjerg, Jackie Snowden, Avideh Shashaani, Harriet Sanford, Dave Trachtenberg and Janine Rudder. And finally, a shout-out to all of our wonderful interns, including Madeleine Sagebiel, whose positive, skillful help was instrumental in the final stages of getting this curriculum to the publisher.

Finally, we are deeply grateful to the funders who make our work possible including The Morris and Gwendolyn Cafritz Foundation, the Bender Foundation, the SuPau Foundation and the Fund for the Future of Our Children, as well as our wonderful corporate and individual donors. We couldn't do it without you!

With love and gratitude,

Linda Ryden and Cheryl Cole Dodwell, August 2021

About Linda Ryden, Teacher and Author

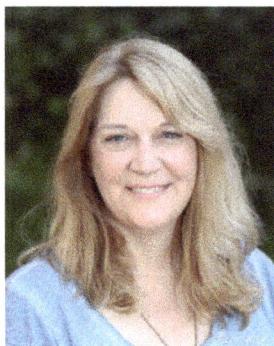

Linda Ryden is the creator of the *Peace of Mind* Program and author of the Peace of Mind Curriculum Series, a cutting-edge combination of mindfulness-based social-emotional learning, conflict resolution and social justice for Early Childhood through Middle School. Linda has served as the full-time Peace Teacher at Lafayette Elementary School, Washington DC's largest public elementary, since 2003 and continues to teach Peace of Mind classes to more than 700 students every week. Linda is also actively engaged in supporting her school's efforts to sustain an inclusive and equitable school climate.

Linda is the author of five mindfulness-based children's books, including three published by Tilbury House. Her work has been featured in *The Washington Post, Washingtonian Magazine, Washington Parent, Washington Family, Teaching Tolerance, Edutopia,* among others. Linda was a keynote speaker at the National Network of State Teachers of the Year conference in 2020 and a featured speaker at the National Education Association Foundation Symposium in 2018, and has received a Commendation for Educational Innovation from the DC Board of Education.

Linda brings a passion for teaching peace and over 25 years of teaching experience to her work with children and adults. Linda lives in Washington D.C. with her husband Jeremiah Cohen, owner of Bullfrog Bagels, their two children, and their dog Phoebe.

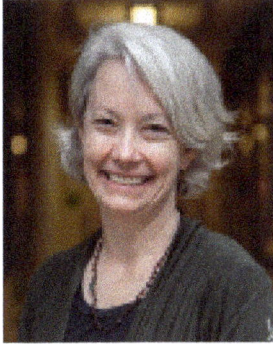

Cheryl Cole Dodwell, the Executive Director of Peace of Mind Inc., is the co-author of the *Peace of Mind Core Curriculum Series* and manages the development of the *Henry and Friends Storybook Series* and all other Peace of Mind resources. Cheryl brings dedication and passion, a love of writing and editing, a background in finance and publishing, education and practice in the management of community organizations, and deep experience in mindfulness, healing practices and parenting to her work with Peace of Mind. She is grateful to be able to contribute to making our world a kinder and inclusive place for all. Cheryl lives in Maryland with her husband James and loves visits from her two kind and inspiring grown up children.

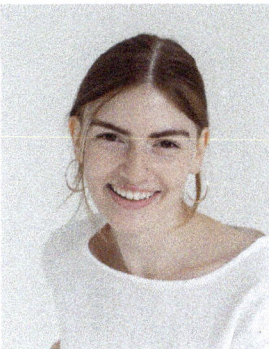

Gigi Gonyea is a textile designer and illustrator. She uses color, pattern and perspective in her designs to create whimsical and joyous spaces. She has a BFA from The Savannah College of Art and Design and a former Peace of Mind student of Linda Ryden.

www.ingramcontent.com/pod-product-compliance
Lightning Source LLC
Chambersburg PA
CBHW042353030426

42336CB00029B/3462